Everything You Need
to Know About

CAREGIVING

for Parkinson's Disease

Everything You Need to Know About
CAREGIVING
for Parkinson's Disease

Lianna Marie

Purdue University Press · West Lafayette, Indiana

For Muriel,
one of the all-time great caregivers

Library of Congress Cataloging-in-Publication Data
Names: Marie, Lianna, 1974– author.
Title: Everything you need to know about caregiving for Parkinson's
    disease / Lianna Marie.
Identifiers: LCCN 2020020344 (print) | LCCN 2020020345
    (ebook) | ISBN 9781557539953 (paperback) | ISBN
    9781557539960 (epub) | ISBN 9781557539977 (pdf)
Subjects: LCSH: Parkinson's disease—Handbooks, manuals, etc. |
    Parkinson's disease—Patients—Care—Handbooks, manuals,
    etc. | Caregivers—Handbooks, manuals, etc.
Classification: LCC RC382 .M3673 2020 (print) | LCC RC382
    (ebook) | DDC 616.8/33—dc23
LC record available at https://lccn.loc.gov/2020020344
LC ebook record available at https://lccn.loc.gov/2020020345

This book is sold with the understanding that neither the author
nor the publisher is engaged in tendering legal, accounting, medical, or other professional advice. If such advice or other assistance is
required, the personal services of a competent professional should
be sought.

Contents

PART 5 GETTING PRACTICAL: CAREGIVING FOR PARKINSON'S

PART 6 ESPECIALLY FOR SPOUSES

PART 7 GETTING HELP

About the Author

A trained nurse, Lianna Marie served as her mother's caregiver and advocate for over 20 years through the many stages of Parkinson's disease. She founded AllAboutParkinsons.com, an online community that has connected and helped thousands of people with the disease, their families, and their caregivers.

The *Complete Guide for People With Parkinson's Disease and Their Loved Ones* is written for people recently diagnosed and their family members; *Everything You Need to Know About Caregiving for Parkinson's Disease* is a go-to resource for all caregivers of those suffering from Parkinson's. Both books share the goal of educating and helping everyday people with no specialized training, providing comprehensive information, practical tips, and guidance about how to deal with the emotional toll of the disease.

Marie speaks frequently to fellow caregivers, guardians, and nurse practitioners. Born and raised near Toronto, Marie now lives with her husband in Seattle. When not writing or speaking, she can be found in the swimming pool, training for her next competition. To learn more about Lianna Marie, her upcoming books, and her speaking schedule, visit www.liannamarie.com.

Also by Lianna Marie

The Complete Guide for People With Parkinson's Disease and Their Loved Ones

The Parkinson's Path: Your Guide to Finding Hope, Happiness, and Meaning on Your Journey With Parkinson's

Fighting Parkinson's: 15 Vital Exercises to Help You Fight the Progression of Parkinson's

How to Parkinson's Proof Your Home: The Essential Guide to Making Your Home Safer for Living With Parkinson's

Find these books and free resources at AllAboutParkinsons.com.

A note from the author

If you enjoy this book or find it helpful, I would be very grateful if you would post a short review where you purchased it. Your support really does make a difference, and I personally read all the reviews.

Preface

My mom lived with Parkinson's for 30 years. She spent the last eight years of her life battling dementia as well, which made for an extra challenging time for those of us who loved and cared for her. If you've experienced dementia with a loved one, I know you understand.

Even though Mom succumbed to dementia, I think most would say it's remarkable that she survived three decades with Parkinson's, given that the average amount time people with this disease have from diagnosis to death is 16 years. I believe it was her faith and determination, as well as the caregivers she had over the years, that made the most significant difference.

Mom was fortunate enough to have a team of people around her that helped make life easier as her illness progressed. I was one of those team members, and my role was hands-on for most of that time, either in her home or in nursing homes in the late stages of her disease. For a few years I cared for Mom long distance and experienced how hard that can be, so I certainly relate to folks who've had to do that for their loved one.

When Mom was in the early stages of PD, she only needed help with simple tasks like getting out of a chair or car seat now and then. Over time, Mom's needs increased and tasks like helping her walk to the bathroom when her wheels (aka legs) were shut down, delivering medications to her at the scheduled times, and taking on household jobs like cooking and cleaning were just a few of the things that I, as well as her other caregivers, took on.

One of Mom's caregivers through the mid-stages of her disease was her husband, Dave. They married in the 10th year of Mom's illness, and he vowed to take care of her "in sickness and in health." Dave took on many of the tasks Mom needed doing, all while trying to maintain a stress-free environment for her so as to minimize her symptoms—an assignment most people would find challenging.

As the years passed, the physical stress and emotional demands of caregiving became too much for Dave, so both he and my mom sought external help. This help took many forms, including care workers who helped them in their home, support groups for both of them, a short-term respite from a care facility, and caregiving from family members like myself.

Unfortunately, throughout his many years of caring for Mom, Dave neglected to take care of himself. He developed diabetes as well as skin and colon cancer. Despite his illnesses, Dave was a loyal and loving caregiver. He visited Mom in the nursing home and took her on outings whenever he was able. He even volunteered and helped raise funds for his local Parkinson's foundation. Sadly, his illnesses became too much for him, and Dave passed away.

I know our story is not unique. Having read hundreds of stories from fellow Parkinson's caregivers, I found that many are doing their utmost for their loved ones with Parkinson's but are finding it overwhelming and sometimes detrimental to their health.

As a caregiver and advocate for my mom, I embarked upon a mission to help her receive the best quality and quantity of care possible. After seeing the toll that caregiving took on Dave and, conversely, what his and my family's efforts did to help improve Mom's quality of life, I feel compelled to help other caregivers care for themselves while caring for their loved one.

I hope this book can be a new chapter in your caregiving journey—one in which you find encouragement and support, as well as practical tips and guidance, to help you navigate the various challenges you may face.

I will finish here with a quote from an interview Mom gave around the 12th year of her journey with Parkinson's. She was speaking about what enabled her to keep going day after day, but I think it applies to us caregivers as well: "Each day we must remind ourselves why we do what we do. We must find meaning in our lives outside of caregiving and focus on the joys and fulfillment we can gain from caring for our loved one."

—*Lianna*

Words You Need to Know

Antioxidant: an enzyme or other organic substance, such as vitamin E or beta-carotene, that is capable of counteracting the damaging effects of oxidation to the cells in the body

Bradykinesia: slowness of movement

Dopamine: a chemical substance (neurotransmitter) found in the brain that sends impulses from one nerve cell to another and helps to regulate movement, balance, attention, learning, and emotional responses; the substance that is lost with Parkinson's

Dopamine agonists: drugs that imitate the effects of dopamine

Dyskinesia: an involuntary movement that can accompany peak doses of levodopa; the most common and disruptive side effect of Parkinson's medications

Dystonia: sustained muscle contractions or cramps that some people with Parkinson's experience

Excessive daytime sleepiness (EDS): a condition that causes people with Parkinson's to fall asleep or doze frequently during normal waking hours

Freezing: when people with advanced Parkinson's have a temporary, involuntary inability to move; sometimes referred to as "FOG," or "freezing of gait"

Levodopa: the most effective antiparkinsonian drug; levodopa is changed into dopamine in the brain and is usually combined with the drug carbidopa and marketed as Sinemet

Neurologist: a specialist in the diagnosis and treatment of disorders of the nervous system (Note: In this book I often use the word doctor instead of neurologist)

On/off time: the cycle that people with Parkinson's go through in relation to their dose of levodopa medication; "on" refers to the time when the medication is working to control symptoms, and "off" refers to when it has worn off and symptoms are poorly controlled; off times are more common as the disease progresses

Parkinsonism: the umbrella term given to a group of neurological disorders that feature Parkinson's movement symptoms such as bradykinesia, tremor, stiffness of muscles, and gait and balance problems

PD: short form for Parkinson's disease

Pill rolling tremor: a typical Parkinson's tremor; it looks like the person is rolling a pill between the thumb and forefinger

PWP: a person with Parkinson's disease

Restless legs syndrome (RLS): an irresistible desire to move the legs and a common cause of sleeplessness in Parkinson's

Tremor: involuntary shaking of the hands, arms, legs, jaw, or tongue

Young-onset Parkinson's disease (YOPD): the diagnosis given to someone aged 21 to 50 years; also known as early onset Parkinson's disease

PART 1

Caregiving Essentials

1. Who Cares?

"I don't consider caring for my Mom a 'job.' Though some days are emotionally draining, it's the least I could do for the person who gave me the wonderful life I've lived. I wouldn't trade the time I've spent with her for the world."

—ANONYMOUS, PARKINSON'S CAREGIVER

When you hear the word caregiver, what you think of will most likely depend on whether you've ever been one. Google may tell you it's merely a person who gives help and protection to someone (such as a child, an older person, or someone who is sick), but what they don't expand on is what that help might look like, practically speaking.

Those of us who have been a caregiver for someone with Parkinson's know you can't sum up our role in one short sentence. Our responsibilities may include helping our loved one with daily tasks such as preparing meals, shopping, housekeeping, and laundry; keeping track of medication schedules and prescriptions; assisting with or being in charge of finances; assisting with bathing, grooming, dressing, toileting, and exercise; taking them to appointments; helping them get in and out of a wheelchair, car, or shower; helping them walk through doorways or cramped spaces; or being their companion, cheerleader, and emotional supporter.

In this book I will be discussing issues specific to those caring for someone with Parkinson's disease and topics that are relevant to caregivers of any kind. Yes, you must understand that regardless of whom you are caring for, many of the problems you will face apply to ALL caregivers. In other words, you are not alone.

You may be surprised to learn just how many caregivers there are in this world. Estimates indicate there are almost 44 million people providing care for a family member or loved one in the United States, 7.8 million in Canada, 6.5 million in the U.K., and

2.7 million in Australia . . . And those are just the countries on which I could find statistics![1]

Here are some quick stats on caregiving in the U.S.[2]

- Nearly 44 million adults are providing personal assistance for family members with disabilities or other care needs.
- 60 percent of caregivers are female.
- The average age of caregivers is 49.
- The typical caregiver has been helping a parent or spouse for four years.
- More than 15 million caregivers provide care for someone with dementia.
- A third of family caregivers say they do it alone, receiving no help from anyone.
- Over one-quarter of caregivers are "sandwiched" between caregiving and raising children.
- 6 in 10 caregivers care for an adult with a long-term physical condition.
- 6 in 10 caregivers are employed.

Caregiving types

There are many types of caregivers; some live in the same house as their loved one, whereas others live miles and miles away. Some are spouses, while others are sons or daughters. Some may even care for a parent while still caring for their own children. When I was my mom's caregiver, I did so both in a live-in situation and while living far away from her.

The following are the main types of caregivers to whom most organizations refer. Note that you may fall into more than one of these categories.

The crisis caregiver: This term applies if your loved one or family member does fine on his or her own until there's an emergency—that's when you step in.

4

The working caregiver: You are taking on a caregiving role (be it physical and/or financial) in addition to holding down a part-time or full-time job.

The sandwich generation caregiver: This term was coined to describe those caregivers who take care of not only their children but their elderly parents too. They are "sandwiched" between two generations.

The spousal caregiver: When a life partner becomes ill, a caregiver must deal with many challenging and sometimes heart-wrenching issues, including adjusting to one's partner becoming the patient, as well as intimacy issues.

The long-distance caregiver: If you live in a different city, state/province, or country than your loved one, you are a long-distance caregiver. Even though they live far away, long-distance caregivers can be responsible for the financial, medical, and personal needs of their loved ones and help them by telephone.

Though the term may sound a bit funny, the sandwich generation caregiver has become so prevalent in our society that both Merriam-Webster and Oxford University Press have added "sandwich generation" to their dictionaries.

2. Before You Say Yes to Caregiving

"Living with Parkinson's disease can be overwhelming. When my husband was first diagnosed, we were both frightened by what lay ahead for us. It was all an uncharted course for us. I made him promise me that he would not give up and that he would cooperate with me as I tried to help him. He has kept that promise, and I believe that it has drawn us closer. We have good days and days when he has a hard time. On the bad days, we just blame 'Parky' for his troubles."

—ANONYMOUS, PARKINSON'S CAREGIVER

Caregiving is a choice. Though as many as half of all caregivers say they never chose their caregiving gig,[3] you need to know that regardless of whether you feel you have a choice, you do.

Before blindly rushing into caregiving, it's a good idea to look at your needs first. Whether you are considering caring for someone with Parkinson's, someone with dementia, or simply an aging parent, caregiving can take a huge toll on both your health and your finances if you're not careful.

Here are three essential questions you should ask yourself before you commit to caregiving.

1. Are you physically and emotionally ready?

Most people who take on the caregiving role aren't prepared for its many challenges and how quickly it takes over your life. The good news is you can make the caregiving journey a more pleasant and rewarding one by readying yourself ahead of time. How? A key factor is to become empowered. Tell yourself you can do this! Face your fears of "not being qualified for the job" and break free of beliefs that may be limiting you.

Another thing you'll want to consider as you contemplate taking on the caregiving role is how it will affect your relationships. If you are married, is your spouse supportive of or negative toward caregiving? If you don't have a spouse or partner, how will this affect your ability to be a caregiver? If you have kids, how will your caregiver role affect them and your relationship with them?

2. Are you financially ready?

Caring for a family member can be expensive and seriously impact a caregiver's finances. As we will discuss in chapter 8, you must plan your finances ahead of time. Additional factors such as whether you have children and the state of your care receiver's funds will also impact your decision as to whether you'll take on the caregiving role.

3. Are you legally ready?

Do you know your loved one's wishes in the end stages of their life? Do they have a plan to pay for their care if need be? Without certain legal documents in place, caring for your loved one can be a lot more challenging than it has to be. You can help your loved one plan for their current and future medical and financial needs by working with them to prepare six essential legal documents. These documents can help make difficult situations easier to navigate. Also, knowing that you're carrying out your loved one's wishes can give you peace of mind and ease the feelings of guilt that many caregivers experience. You can read more about these essential legal and financial documents in chapter 9.

4. Can you say no to caregiving?

Maybe you've taken an honest look at your ability and willingness to commit to being a caregiver and are feeling that it's not right for you. If that's the case and you're looking for permission to say no to caregiving, no one is going to give it to you—except you. You may think, "But I can't say no to Mom. She was always there for me growing up; how could I NOT be there for her now?" Rest easy. Caregiving isn't for everyone. Though it's tough saying no to your loved one, sometimes it's the less selfish, more loving, and more caring thing to do.

Passing the role onto another family member or a professional can save you from burning out and may even strengthen your relationship with your loved one if it's done with love and honesty.

In my case, I don't know if there was ever a question as to whether I would care for my mom—it was more a question of how I could best care for her. Early on, I learned that supporting my stepdad (Mom's primary caregiver at the time) was the best way for me to care for her. Then, as her care needs became more significant and it became apparent that my stepdad was getting burned out, I became more involved in Mom's care.

Years later, my family (in consultation with my mom and stepdad) decided to move her to a care facility. This helped take the burden off all of us while allowing her to get the care she needed. I don't consider this to have been us saying no to caregiving, but rather us making a choice to care for her in a different way.

There is no right or wrong when it comes to the decision of caregiving. Everyone is different and you have to make the choices that are best for you.

It's important to note that the effects of caregiving are not all negative. Many surveys suggest that, for some, caregiving builds confidence, teaches them how to deal with difficult situations, brings them closer to their loved one, and gives them the satisfaction of knowing that their loved one is getting the quality of care they desire.[4]

3. Get Help

"The number one best advice I think is to get into a support group. You realize that you are not alone, and that goes for both the Parkinsonian and their caregiver."

—MARY S., PARKINSON'S CAREGIVER

As you know, Parkinson's disease is a chronic disorder that causes a wide variety of motor and nonmotor symptoms. Because the disease is progressive, the risk of complications such as falls and loss of independence can have a big impact on the quality of life of your loved one.

Doctors and researchers have found that having a multidisciplinary approach to treating Parkinson's is the best way to improve the lives of people with the disease. The team approach can also reduce hospitalizations and save money.

As a caregiver, you are a vital member of your loved one's Parkinson's care team. But you can't—and shouldn't try—to carry all the weight yourself. By knowing all the team members that can help your loved one, you may be able to direct certain aspects of their care to one or more of them.

Team members for people with Parkinson's include the neurologist (for periodic disease checkups and medication adjustments), family physician (for regular check-ups and tests, as well as help with secondary PD symptoms such as constipation and sleep issues), certified dietician or nutritionist (to ensure they are eating the right foods for their medications to be most effective), occupational therapist (to suggest assistive devices and train your loved one in their use), speech therapist (for problems with speaking and swallowing), massage therapist (to relieve pain that often accompanies PD), gastroenterologist (for those with constipation or other gastrointestinal issues), ophthalmologist (for vision problems, including double vision, which can occur in PD), mental health specialist (for depression and/or anxiety, which often accompanies PD), and physical therapist (to help retrain muscles and keep your loved one moving).

In addition to the aforementioned Parkinson's team members, it's important that you find all the other support and respite resources that are available to you. Though you may not need the help now, gathering a list of people and organizations who can help you and your loved one will save you time and effort down the road and prove to be a lifesaver.

Here are just a few of the places and people to which family caregivers can turn for help.

- Family, friends, and neighbors
- Online forums and Facebook (FB) groups (look for All About Parkinson's on FB)
- Local support groups (ask about them through your local PD association)
- Church or outreach groups that serve those in need
- Local home care organizations
- Local and national Parkinson's associations
- Local and national Alzheimer's associations
- Local and national administrations on aging

You can read more about how and where to get help in chapters 40–44.

If you or your loved one is considering attending a support group (for caregivers or for people with Parkinson's), make sure you call the moderator ahead of time to find out more about the group's dynamics. It's always good to know who will be in the group so that you can make sure you or your loved one's needs will be met.

4. Set Boundaries

"If caregivers have no boundaries and just blindly do whatever is asked of them at all times, they may burn out before they know what's happening." —ANONYMOUS, PARKINSON'S CAREGIVER

It's not uncommon for caregivers to have challenges setting limits. It's easy to fall into a pattern of saying yes to just about everything your loved one asks you to do. Many say yes before thinking about what might be involved or what they might be committing to.

There are many possible reasons we caregivers do this: we love our spouse or parent so much and don't want to disappoint them; we love being needed; we are a helper-type person and like to fix problems; we feel responsible for the happiness of our loved one; we feel guilty if we say no; we don't want to be seen as neglectful, or we think we're superwoman and should be able to do everything.

Though these are all noble reasons for not setting limits, if you want to make it in this caregiving journey, it is essential that you carefully examine your life and set clear boundaries. In setting these boundaries, you may have to put limits on your time, money, space, or strength. Doing this will make you a stronger caregiver, one who can recover from or adjust easily to hardships or change.

Having boundaries in place that work for everyone can help caregivers continue to care while showing love and concern without feeling desperate, enabling their loved one, or trying to rescue, fix, or control them.

The following strategies can help you set boundaries.

Evaluate

Early in your caregiving journey, have an honest talk with yourself. Think about how much of a commitment you are willing and able to make, and what you can and will do. Remember, caregiving is a team effort with your loved one. Once you have things clear in your mind, have a family meeting to let them know what your boundaries are before problems arise.

Prioritize

Try to remember that caregiving is just ONE component of your life. Decide what matters most in your life and how you want to live out the rest of it. Do you want to maintain your career? How do you envision your marriage 5 or 10 years from now? Those who learn how to manage their personal lives end up being the best caregivers.

Know their limitations

Evaluate your loved one's limitations in relation to other available resources (friends, neighbors, paid help, etc.). Even though you may not always accept all of your loved one's requests, let them know that you care about them. As much as you can, try to help your loved one maintain their independence, as this will keep them happier and healthier longer.

Accept your limitations

We want to provide for all of our loved one's needs, but it's almost impossible to do so. Stick to helping only in areas that you can manage positively. Giving help grudgingly will only leave you both angry and frustrated.

Stick to your decisions

If your loved one asks you to do something that you consider unreasonable or simply more than you can manage, explain your position and suggest alternatives. Some people have trouble accepting the losses that can accompany Parkinson's, but as tough as it sometimes may be, you need to remember that you're not responsible for your loved one's happiness.

Detach

You might think this sounds cold and unloving, but it's not. Detaching simply means living a life that isn't centered on someone else's. It is the ability to be close to your loved one without giving up your independence.

To be detached is to recognize your loved one's anger or frustration without taking it personally in terms of something you did or didn't do. It's avoiding jumping in right away to fix a complaint and instead expressing interest and asking them to offer solutions.

You can detach by making caregiving a smaller part of your life. Focus on personal fulfillment through hobbies, relationships, volunteering, getting active, or learning new things.

Give yourself a break

What motivates you to be a caregiver? Think about why you took on the role. Decide to make it something you chose, not something forced on you. Stay connected to your friends and family and the things that make you happy. Laugh and cry often, and be gentle when judging yourself. Most of all, try not to take yourself too seriously!

> If you are caring for a spouse with PD, it's especially important that you learn to set boundaries. You can read about the specific challenges of spousal caregivers and strategies to deal with them in chapters 35–39.

5. Take Care of Yourself

"Have frequent breaks from looking after them. You need some-body else to support you by taking over from time to time. If you get tired and stressed, you won't be much use to the sufferer, so you have to look after yourself as well."

—CAMILLA, PARKINSON'S CAREGIVER

Whether you're new to caregiving of you've been a caregiver for many years, you've probably read or heard the oxygen mask story. If you haven't heard this analogy before, let me quickly explain.

When you fly on a plane there's a mandatory safety briefing you receive from the flight attendants prior to takeoff. The briefing isn't that exciting, but it contains a very important instruction: "In the event of a change in air pressure, put on your own oxygen mask before assisting others."

When you hear this for the first time, your immediate response is, "No way; I need to take care of my kids (husband, mom, best friend, etc.) first!" The idea opposes your instincts. The problem with this thinking is that if you don't put on your mask first, you won't be there for those who need you—you'll be unconscious.

The same instruction applies to caregivers. Because we love and care so much, we often focus all our attention on our loved one and neglect to take care of ourselves. However, just like with the oxygen mask, we need to take care of ourselves so that we can effectively take care of our loved ones.

Following are some tips to help you take better care of yourself.

Decide that your life matters

It's easy to become consumed with caring for your loved one, even to the point of feeling like you have to be on call all the time. You must realize that you deserve time to yourself to regain peace and calm in your life.

14

Deciding that your life matters just as much as your loved one's is the first step toward taking better care of yourself and making the most of your time away from them.

Take responsibility for your care

You can't control Parkinson's and how it will affect your loved one. You can, however, take control of your care. Contrary to what you might think, focusing on your needs while being a caregiver is not selfish—it's an essential part of the job. Don't forget: YOU are responsible for taking care of yourself.

There are many things you can do to take control of your care.

- Make sure you're getting enough rest.
- Pay attention to your nutrition (eating crappy food makes you feel crappy).
- Exercise regularly (even if it's for only 15 minutes at a time).
- Learn to look for and accept other people's help and support.
- Learn and use stress-reduction techniques (e.g., meditation, prayer, yoga, tai chi).
- Take time off (without feeling guilty).
- Find ways to nurture your body and soul (e.g., take a hot bath; read a good book).
- Talk to a friend, counselor, or pastor about your feelings when you need to.
- Reduce negativity in your life.

Reduce your stress levels

Several factors influence stress levels in any caregiving situation. Stress is not just affected by the situation itself, but also by how you perceive it. For example, some naturally see the glass as half full while others see it as half empty. Remembering that you're not the only one in this situation may help you see and cope with things differently.

Other factors may influence your stress levels. One is whether your caregiving job was voluntary. If you feel that you had no choice in taking on the responsibility, it's more likely that you'll feel resentful toward your loved one and experience tension in your relationship. Another is the amount of care your loved one needs. For instance, caring for someone with dementia is often more stressful than caring for someone who has only physical limitations. And your stress levels *will* be increased if you have little to no support.

Reducing your stress levels is possible by learning stress-reduction techniques (described in detail in chapter 11). As you're doing this, think about how you have coped with stress in the past.

Set goals

Setting goals is a key part of taking care of yourself. If you've never set goals before, think of it simply as writing a list of things you want to get done. Start with a list of things you would like to accomplish in the next month, then three months, then six months. Set small and big goals. Break the big goals down into smaller action steps. This will increase your likelihood of accomplishing them. Also, the more specific you can be with your goals, the better.

Here are some examples of goals you might set.

- Take a two-week vacation from caregiving.
- Get help from a community organization for caregiving tasks.
- Exercise three times a week for 30 minutes each time.
- Work on a new hobby or job idea for 5 hours a week.

Get rid of negativity

There's enough negativity in this world; you don't need to add to it by being negative toward yourself. Negative self-talk is another barrier to caring for yourself and achieving your goals. Saying things to yourself like "I can never find the time to do the things I want," or "I can never do anything right" is counterproductive and can cause unnecessary anxiety. Instead, try talking positively to yourself. Use the words "I can do . . ." and "I'm good at . . ." to start your sentences. Remember, your mind is very powerful and believes what you tell it.

Identify personal barriers

Do you find it easier to take care of others than to take care of yourself? If this has been your pattern, you may have beliefs and personal barriers standing in the way of your taking care of yourself. If that's the case, ask yourself: What good will I be to my loved one if I get sick or, even worse, if I die?

Breaking old patterns can be challenging, but it can be done. It doesn't matter what caregiving situation you're in or how long you've been in it. The first step in removing personal barriers to caring for yourself is to identify what is in your way. Try asking yourself these questions.

- Do I think I'm selfish if I put my needs first?
- Do I have trouble asking for what I need, or do I feel like a failure if I do?
- Do I do too much because I feel as though I have to prove that I'm worthy of my loved one's affection?

Another barrier that can get in the way of proper self-care is having misconceptions about caregiving. See if you identify with any of these statements.

- I am responsible for my mom's/dad's health.
- If I don't do it, no one will.
- If I do it right, I will get the love, attention, and respect I deserve.
- I promised my mom that I would always take care of my dad.

Beliefs or misconceptions like these can cause caregivers to continually try to do what can't be done and control what can't be controlled. This leads to frustration and feelings of being a failure, which themselves lead to a lack of self-care. If you're not taking good care of yourself, ask yourself what barriers you have put up.

PART 2

What to Expect

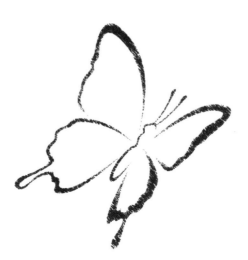

6. How Long Will My Caregiving Role Last?

"It has been a rather unique experience to go from daughter to caregiver of my dad. On the downside, it saddens me to see my dad need help. On the upside, I have become reacquainted with my dad, his personality, and his sense of humor."

—ANONYMOUS, PARKINSON'S CAREGIVER

One of the many questions you may be asking yourself as a caregiver is how long your role will last. This is a tough question to answer because, as you've probably already heard, Parkinson's varies from person to person so it's impossible to say how long you will be taking on your caregiving role.

Statistics say the average length of time spent as a caregiver of any kind is about four years.[5] For those caring for someone with Parkinson's, the time you spend will depend on what stage your loved one was in when you took over your caregiving role.

In most cases, Parkinson's disease progresses slowly, and, on average, people with PD live between 10 and 20 years after diagnosis. Factors such as being diagnosed later in life, scoring poorly on movement tests, experiencing delusions, hallucinations, or other psychotic symptoms, and developing dementia have all been associated with a shorter life expectancy.

The fact is, if you decide to care for your loved one through the end stages of Parkinson's (and not move them into a full-time care facility), you will most likely be facing a caregiving journey of several years.

7. The Physical Side of Caregiving

"My sister was diagnosed with Parkinson's when she was 55 years old. We are learning more and more about it all the time. One thing we both feel is important is to know the symptoms of Parkinson's and to check with a competent doctor. My sister hid her symptoms from all of us for several years. She thought her problems were due to getting older and gaining weight. She noticed a tremor in one hand, had problems getting up from a chair, and could hardly dress herself. Now, with treatment, she dresses herself, goes up and down stairs easily, uses her treadmill regularly, and generally feels much better."

—BARBARA, PARKINSON'S CAREGIVER

About 1 in 10 caregivers report that caregiving has caused their physical health to worsen.[6]

Providing this statistic here isn't meant to scare you away from caregiving but to make you aware of the possible negative impact caregiving can have on your health, especially if you don't learn proper stress management and other coping techniques.

Caregiving can have all the features of a chronic stress experience. In other words, it creates physical and psychological strain over extended periods, is often uncontrollable and unpredictable, often creates secondary stress in other areas of your life (such as your work or relationships), and often requires you to be on high alert. Not all stress is bad for you, but long-term stress of any kind is, and it can lead to serious health problems.

Some of the ways the stress of caregiving can affect your physical health are by weakening your immune system (causing you to get more colds and illnesses than non-caregivers); increasing your risk of chronic illnesses such as heart disease, cancer, arthritis, and diabetes; increasing your susceptibility to depression and anxiety (especially in women); causing you to gain weight (more often in women), sometimes to the point of obesity.

The last point of weight gain is something I'm going to focus on because I've heard from many readers that it is an issue. When I first found out that caregiver weight gain was a "thing," I was quite relieved. Maybe then I could blame the extra 10 to 15 pounds I'd been carrying around on my caring for my mom. Gaining 10 or even 20 pounds is very common for people while they're on a caregiving journey. The stress of it all can lead to emotional eating and poor food choices.

I know I've been guilty of stress and emotional eating in general, and more so when I was caring for Mom. Sometimes I'd grab junk food or overeat without thinking about it. Even though I knew better, unless it was convenient and tasty (no offense to the tofu lovers out there, but sometimes I need a bit more zing to my food) I often cut corners in the "nutritional eating" department.

One thing that helped me get better at this was simply paying more attention to my food choices. I also paid closer attention to portion size, especially on days when I wasn't able to get in my swim workout. Another step I took to ensure that I got all the nutrients I needed was to start taking a multivitamin every day.

Here are some more tips to help lessen caregiver weight gain.

- Plan ahead. The easiest way to eat healthier is to prepare healthy snacks ahead of time. Chop up fresh fruit and veggies and keep them in a Ziploc bag in the fridge (or, even better, save time and buy them prechopped!). You can also buy nuts (e.g., walnuts, almonds, cashews), which are great good-for-you snacks on the go. Another quick, healthy snack is air-popped popcorn.
- Eat for energy. Think of your body as a car that needs fuel. If you regularly fill your tank with junk and processed foods (aka empty calories), you can't expect your engine to perform at its best. Instead, choose foods that will keep your blood sugar stable and provide lots of energy. These include lean protein at every meal, whole grains (e.g., oats),

foods high in omega-3 fatty acids (e.g., salmon), and lots of plants, including fruits, vegetables, and nuts.

- Stick to simple recipes with minimal ingredients to get meals onto your plate sooner. For example, for dinner you could pan-fry a chicken breast, heat some frozen vegetables, and make five-minute brown rice.
- When you cook, make enough for leftovers to have the next day, or freeze them for another time when you need a quick meal.
- Pay attention to what you're eating. Avoid multitasking during mealtime so that you can taste and enjoy your food, as well as pay attention to portion sizes.
- Get help from friends and family to prepare your snacks or bring over dinner when you feel overwhelmed.
- Don't self-medicate with alcohol. It's okay to enjoy your wine, but make sure you're not using alcohol as a crutch. I am a red wine lover, but moderation is essential for me to maintain a healthy weight.
- If cooking for yourself and your loved one is becoming more and more difficult, consider home-delivered meal services. Your loved one may qualify to get these paid for by a government program, so it's a good idea to look into that.
- Try premade nutritional shakes when you have to skip a meal.
- Don't forbid yourself to eat yummy, comforting foods like chocolate. It's okay to have this from time to time, just watch how much you eat—moderation is key.
- If you have a sweet tooth like I do, try lower fat/lower sugar alternatives like gelato instead of ice cream. In the summer, try fresh berries on top of angel food cake instead of heavier, more calorically dense cheesecake.
- Strive to reduce your intake of high-sugar, high-fat foods, but don't eliminate all fat. Olive oil, flaxseed oil, and the oil in nuts and fish such as salmon are considered healthy fats.

One of my favorite "good fat" foods is avocado. I eat one of these almost every day on my salad. Homemade guacamole is also a tasty treat!

- If you're taking medications, find out if any of them interact with the food you're eating, as that may cause weight gain. You can ask your doctor or pharmacist about this. Also check out the U.S. National Library of Medicine's Medline-Plus website for detailed info: https://medlineplus.gov/.
- Don't forget that exercising every day can help with maintaining weight. Just remember: you can never out-exercise a bad diet!

If you are experiencing any of the adverse physical effects of caregiver stress, talk to your doctor. It's crucial for you to get the help you need to help prevent any significant health problems.

8. The Costs of Caregiving

"Try and reduce stress in your everyday living by altering your lifestyle. Downsize your home, thus making more money available to you because of the reduced costs of heating bills, electricity, rates, taxes, and maintenance. Invest the savings to increase your income. Better still, move somewhere with a nice climate and lower cost of living. Somewhere dry and sunny and not too humid. If you suffer from rheumatism, you will feel better in that environment. There may come a time when you need help and you will be better prepared to pay the costs."

—REGINALD, PWP

For many, care decisions are driven by the "how much is this going to cost us" question. Whether it be your finances, time, job, or health, you must weigh the various costs of caregiving to ensure you are making the best decisions for yourself and your loved ones.

When it comes to the financial cost of caregiving, many feel their decisions are made for them based on what kind of care (if any) they can afford. For example, had my mom lived outside of Canada, I know we would have had to make different care decisions for her in the late stages of PD as her finances wouldn't have afforded her much time in a care facility in, for example, the U.S.

Being aware of what individual caregiving costs are in your area is very important so that you can make better decisions and plans for yourself and your loved one. The out-of-pocket expenses of caregiving can add up. Many working caregivers end up using all or most of their savings and retirement funds. For those who are considering full-time caregiving, you must understand the financial position you may be getting yourself into down the road.

In addition to the financial costs, one of the greatest hidden costs of caregiving is time. Most people underestimate how much time they will spend providing care. They picture themselves caring for a few hours a week for a couple of months but end up providing care a few hours a day for a couple of (or more) years. Caring.com's 2017 survey found almost 40 percent of caregivers spend more than 30 hours per week caring for their loved one.[7]

By devoting more and more time to their loved ones, caregivers may lose more than just time. Caregivers often must reduce their working hours, leave their jobs temporarily, or take early retirement. Leaving the workforce for a couple of months might be feasible, but doing so for a couple of years could put you in a tight spot financially. A study by MetLife found that the average caregiver's lost wages are $143,000.[8]

For those who leave the workforce to become a caregiver, returning can be a challenge. Many caregivers find it very difficult to get another job after having been away for many months or years.

Your health can be a cost you may not think of when you enter the world of caregiving. Studies have found that many caregivers say their role has caused their own mental and physical health to decline. Researchers have also found that caregivers have worse physical and emotional health than do non-caregivers. This equates to increased health care costs for caregivers, especially those who have lost their health insurance as a result of having left their job to become a caregiver.[9]

The hard costs of caregiving

Though the costs may at first appear to be higher, there are a range of options that can provide the care your loved one needs without costing you time, lost wages, and so forth. Following are the 2019 U.S. national median daily, monthly, and annual rates paid for various types of adult care.[10]

Nursing home (private room): $280/day, $8,517/month, $102,200/year

Nursing home (semi-private room): $247/day, $7,513/month, $90,155/year

Assisted living (private, 1 bedroom): $133/day, $4,051/month, $48,612/year

Home health aide: $144/day, $4,385/month, $52,624/year
Homemaker services: $141/day, $4,290/month, $51,480/year
Adult day health care: $75/day, $1,625/month, $19,500/year

Note: To find costs specific to your state, see the *Genworth Cost of Care Survey 2019* at https://pro.genworth.com/riiproweb /productinfo/pdf/282102.pdf.

> If you're looking for ways to cover the costs of caregiving, check out chapter 43, which includes tips and resources for monetary support.

9. Planning for Parkinson's

"A living will and discussion early in the process really helped us to make decisions that would have been impossible later on as she wasn't able to answer for herself. It helped us to let her pass with no regrets, no trips to the hospital just because, and no rest home. And most importantly, we, her children, knew exactly what she would want. Hospice was a Godsend and with the living will there was no question we were doing the things that my mother wanted." —ANONYMOUS, PARKINSON'S CAREGIVER

Many people go into caregiving without giving it much thought. They see their loved one in need, so they help. Rarely do they stop and think that their caregiving job could go on for years or that maybe they should plan things out.

Planning is vital for all caregivers, but especially for those caring for someone with Parkinson's. This disease is unpredictable, meaning no two days are the same, nor are any two cases of PD the same. Once you've decided to take on the role of caregiver, you must understand that the care needs of your loved one can change daily. Because of this, it's essential for you to learn how to plan so that you are able to adapt to unexpected changes in your loved one's health and care needs. Planning is also necessary so you don't undermine your health while caring for your loved one.

Here are four key things you'll want to do after you've decided to say yes to caregiving.

1. Get organized

When it comes to caring for people with Parkinson's, the importance of planning and being organized cannot be overemphasized. Without the right legal and financial documentation, you and your loved one could face many problems in an emergency.

Doctors may refuse to discuss important medical information with you, and your loved one may not get the end-of-life care they desire. Also, if your loved one becomes incapacitated, control over their bank accounts and property could be given to a complete stranger.

You can help your loved one plan for their current and future medical and financial needs by working with them to prepare six essential legal documents: a HIPAA authorization, health care power of attorney (POA), living will/advance healthcare directive, financial POA, trust, and will. Detailed descriptions of these six documents are included at the end of this chapter.

2. Be prepared for an emergency

In the event of an emergency, there are a few things you can have ready ahead of time to save yourself from panic.

- Keep a record of your loved one's doctor's office hours, including separate walk-in hours if applicable.
- Write down the location and phone numbers of the closest and highest-rated emergency rooms and urgent care clinics.
- Have a list of your loved one's allergies, medications, medical conditions, and blood type handy.
- Keep copies of health insurance cards and/or policy information.
- Make copies of legal medical documents (HIPAA, health care POA, living will/advance health care directive).
- Keep a record of your loved one's surgeries and tests (including dates and hospital locations).

3. Make a financial plan

Caring for a family member can make a severe dent in your finances. A recent survey found that over 60 percent of family caregivers say they have no plan as to how they will pay for their parents' care over the next five years.[11]

Even with the help of government-funded programs, caregivers often spend tens of thousands of dollars out of their own pockets to cover the medical costs of caring for their loved ones in their last five years of life. For this reason, it's so important that you take steps to secure your personal finances as soon as you possibly can and keep your future long-term care needs in mind.

Here are a few ways to manage your money while caregiving. These may apply to both the caregiver and care receiver.

- Maximize your employer benefit programs (for working caregivers).
- Consider purchasing long-term care insurance.
- Appoint someone to be your financial and health care power of attorney.
- Ensure that you have a current will.
- Make sure you have the life, property, and casualty insurance coverage that meets your needs.

4. Reach out for help

Caregiving is hard work, and you should never underestimate how mentally and emotionally exhausting it can be. Getting help is not just a good idea but essential if you expect to maintain your role as a caregiver for any length of time. Support can come from many people, including friends, family, neighbors, and respite workers from local organizations.

* * *

Here are the six essential legal documents to have ready for your loved one.

MEDICAL DOCUMENTS

1. HIPAA authorization (U.S. only)

The Health Information Portability and Accountability Act (HIPAA) was created to protect the privacy of a patient's health information. Under this law, doctors and other medical professionals, as well as caregivers, are not allowed to discuss a patient's health information with anyone but the patient, unless the patient has provided them with a HIPAA release form. Your loved one can get a copy of this document at their doctor's office.

2. Health care power of attorney (POA)

A health care POA gives legal permission for a trusted person (e.g., a family member, friend, or caregiver) to make healthcare decisions on your behalf. This document would allow a person with PD, for example, to grant legal authority to a trusted relative or friend to make healthcare decisions on their behalf. The person with health care POA could then determine things like where the person with PD lives, what they eat, who bathes them, and what medical care they receive.

Note: There can be some confusion when it comes to the difference between "durable" and "nondurable" powers of attorney. A durable POA is a document that stays in effect indefinitely—either until a person dies or until they recover sufficiently to regain control over their affairs. A nondurable POA terminates either when a person become incapacitated or on a fixed date specified in the document.

3. Living will or advance health care directive

LIVING WILL

A living will, also known in some places as a health care declaration, lets a person state what type of medical treatment they do or do not wish to receive if they are no longer able to make decisions for themselves because of illness or incapacity. Basically, it is a document that speaks for the person when the person is not able to do so.

A living will outlines how a person wants their end-of-life care managed (i.e., aggressive medical care versus hospice care) and may also include a do not resuscitate (DNR) order or an instruction not to insert a feeding tube if they become incapable of eating on their own.

ADVANCE DIRECTIVE

The term "advance directive" usually refers to a single legal document that combines a living will/health care declaration and a durable health care POA. It is currently used in most states in the U.S. Technically, however, both living wills and durable POAs for health care are types of advance directives.

The advance directive provides your loved one with many more options, including the naming of a health care agent. With the advance directive, your loved one can also make decisions ahead of time about life-sustaining procedures in the event that they become incapacitated or are too ill to do so for themselves.

If your loved one has prepared an advance directive or living will, you should review it from time to time and update their directions if their wishes relating to health care have changed. Also, new medical treatments might become available that could impact their health care decisions.

A good online resource to help you with creating an advance directive can be found at Davis Phinney Foundation for Parkinson's (https://www.davisphinneyfoundation.org/blog/advance-directives -and-parkinsons/).

FINANCIAL DOCUMENTS

4. Financial power of attorney (POA)

A financial POA gives a trusted person (i.e., a family member, friend, or caregiver) the authority to act on behalf of the care receiver to make legally binding decisions in their financial matters. An individual with financial POA has the authority to manage a person's finances, which may include paying bills, liquidating assets to cover expenses, and making other investment decisions.

If the care receiver doesn't have the energy, desire, or ability to deal with financial matters, this document will allow someone else to do it for them.

It's important to note that by granting a financial POA, a person doesn't give up their power over their financial affairs; they simply delegate a representative who can sign documents, write checks, or sell real estate for them.

5. Trust

A trust is a legal document that lets a person put conditions on how specific assets will be distributed when they die. Trusts can also help minimize gift and estate taxes. The main difference between a trust and a will is that a trust takes effect as soon as it is created, whereas a will goes into effect only after the person dies.

Another difference between a trust and a will is that a will goes through probate, meaning a court looks at the will and makes sure it gets distributed the way it was written to be. A trust doesn't go through probate and, unlike a will that becomes part of the public record, it can remain private.

A trust does not replace a will. Most trusts deal only with specific assets, such as life insurance or a piece of property, while a will governs the distribution of nearly everything else in the estate.

6. Will

A will is a legal document that directs who will receive a person's assets and property after they die. It also appoints a legal representative to carry out their wishes. Wills and trusts each have their advantages and disadvantages. For example, a will lets a person specify funeral arrangements and name a guardian for children, but a trust doesn't. Conversely, a trust can be used to plan for disability or save money on taxes. An elder law attorney can advise your loved one on the best ways to use a will and a trust in their estate plan.

> If getting all these documents together makes you feel overwhelmed, don't worry! An elder law attorney can guide you through the process. For more information see https://www.naela.org/.

PART 3

The Emotional Side of Caregiving

10. What to Do When You Feel Overwhelmed

"Keep on truckin' until the end." —MY MOM, VAL, PWP

If you're feeling overwhelmed with caregiving, you're not alone. It's common to feel like you're in over your head in terms of managing the stress, worries, new skills, and piles of details involved in caring for another person.

I felt this emotion several times during my caregiving journey with my mom, and I'd like to think that each time I did I got a little bit better at handling it. The reality is there's a learning curve in caregiving. When you start, you might imagine that every other caregiver out there has got it all together, but that's simply not true. Everyone struggles with different aspects of caregiving and has moments when they feel their life is falling apart. It's learning how to get through these struggles that makes your journey more manageable and even rewarding.

Here are a few things you can do when you find yourself feeling overwhelmed.

- Don't look at everything all at once. Remember the mantra "One day (or hour) at a time." Break your tasks into daily and weekly chunks and try not to look too much further than a month down the road. Don't make your to-do lists too long or arduous; you'll feel like you're accomplishing more when you are able to cross multiple small things off your list.
- Put together a team. Remember what I said before about the importance of having a team to help your loved one and his or her evolving needs. Figure out who can help, whom you can trust, and whom you are comfortable asking for what you need. If you can spread the burdens

of decision-making, hands-on care, household maintenance, and so on, it's less on you. Don't be shy about
reaching out.

- Don't aim for perfection. Remember that you're not superwoman (or man) and that you shouldn't try to be. If you
always aim for the impossible, you'll always feel like you've
failed. Instead, aim to do a pretty darn good job and you'll
have better success at reaching your goal.

- Know that you will mess up from time to time, and forgive
yourself when you do. Remember: each day is a new start!

- Find out ways to be prepared for the biggest issues
related to your loved one's Parkinson's so you can be
ready for them.

11. How to Manage Caregiver Stress and Prevent Burnout

"My husband has PD and we've learned that laughter makes a world of difference for everyone involved. He downloads podcasts of the public radio program called *Wait, Wait Don't Tell Me!* and listens to it in the car. It's a great show for creating real belly laughs." —CHRIS M., PARKINSON'S CAREGIVER

It seems everyone has something to be stressed about these days. Stress is becoming so prevalent in people's lives that you may not feel normal if you aren't stressing about something.

As a caregiver, many of the feelings you'll feel are normal, but caregiver stress can be a real problem, and if it's not managed, it can lead to burnout. Also, if that isn't enough reason to take care of your stress levels, keep in mind that caregivers experiencing extreme stress may age prematurely.[12]

Stress is not just an issue for you as a caregiver, but also for your loved one with Parkinson's. It's true: stress can have a very negative impact on the symptoms of Parkinson's disease, especially tremor and mobility. This makes it even more critical for you to learn ways to control and manage your stress levels, as your actions affect not only your health but that of your loved one as well.

It's a real-life scenario. You get stressed out from your caregiving duties, which then makes your loved one stressed out, causing them to lose mobility, which leads to both of you being more stressed out, and so on.

If you're unsure whether you have caregiver stress, here are some common symptoms to look for.

- Depression
- Withdrawal
- Anxiety

- Insomnia
- Anger
- Exhaustion
- Headaches
- Excess perspiration
- Chest pain
- Hair loss
- Trouble concentrating
- Nervous habits like chain-smoking
- Increased use of alcohol or stimulants
- Changes in appetite
- Back, shoulder, or neck pain; muscle tension
- Weight fluctuation (gain or loss)
- High blood pressure, irregular heartbeat, palpitations
- Skin disorders (hives, eczema, psoriasis, tics, itching)
- Periodontal disease, jaw pain
- Reproductive problems/infertility
- Sexual dysfunction/lack of libido
- Weakened immune system (getting more colds, flu, infections)
- Stomach/digestive problems (upset or acid stomach, cramps, heartburn, gas, irritable bowel syndrome, constipation, diarrhea)

As mentioned previously, if you don't manage caregiver stress, it can lead to burnout. Hopefully your stress levels will never get you to the point of exhaustion, but if they do, you must be able to identify that you're in that state so you can get the help you need.

So, how do you know if you're burned out? The short answer is that you will be physically, mentally, and emotionally exhausted. Burnout can happen for several reasons, mostly from not getting the help you need or from trying to do more than you are physically or financially able to.

Signs of caregiver burnout include all those of caregiver stress but also include the following.

- Feeling helpless or hopeless
- Feeling exhausted all the time
- Feeling increasingly resentful
- Being unable to relax
- Being on the verge of tears or crying a lot
- Getting upset over little things
- Being short-tempered with your loved one frequently
- Losing interest in your work
- Increasing use of medications for sleeplessness, anxiety, depression
- Increasing thoughts of death

The following strategies can help you manage stress and prevent burnout. Not all techniques work for everyone, so you may have to experiment a little to find something that works for you. Remember that the key to successful stress management is practice.

Prioritize your to-do list

If you're like most caregivers, your to-do lists can get pretty long and cumbersome. Accept that you can't always get everything done in one day. Prioritize your lists, set up a daily routine, and break large tasks into small doable chunks to help you get more things done.

Say no

Many people (including me) have a fear of missing out on things, so they say yes to events that end up taking more energy than they are worth. Say no to social requests that are draining or stressful (e.g., hosting holiday get-togethers). Knowing your limits and what you can handle is essential so that you don't overextend yourself.

Practice deep breathing

Take slow, deep breaths from your diaphragm. Breathe in through your nose and out through your mouth. Count to five as you breathe in and five as you breathe out. Do this several times until you begin to feel more relaxed.

Try progressive relaxation

Here's a quick and easy way to calm your mind if you feel stressed: Get in a comfortable position, close your eyes, and slowly focus on relaxing different parts of your body, one at a time. Start at your head and work your way down to your feet.

If you need some help, there is a booming industry of smart-phone apps that can guide you.

Relax with music

There are many benefits to listening to music, including relaxation and pain management. You can find all kinds of relaxation materials in bookstores and music stores or on the Internet. You may have to experiment a little to find something that works for you. I find listening to my favorite spa music with noise-canceling headphones to be a great way to escape the noise of the world.

Music is useful not only for you but also for the person with Parkinson's, making it easier to work with them. We used music as much as possible to get Mom going when she was stuck somewhere, as well as to lift her mood when she was in a funk.

Whether we had her hooked up to an iPod, had her favorite music playing on a stereo, or were humming a marching tune loudly along beside her, it was incredible to watch how she could go from being completely immobile to practically running across the room!

Meditate or pray

Did you know that both meditation and prayer have scientifically proven health benefits? When you meditate or pray, the activity of your brain moves from the right frontal cortex (where stress lives) to the calm left frontal cortex. This results in feeling relaxed, which then slows down your breathing. When your breathing slows to 6 to 10 breaths a minute, your breath becomes aligned with the rhythms in your heart, which is good for your cardiovascular health.[13]

Other physical benefits of meditation and prayer include decreased blood pressure, deep rest, and easier breathing. Some mental benefits include greater creativity, reduced anxiety and depression, improved learning and memory, and increased happiness and emotional stability.

Pamper yourself

Set aside time to treat yourself to something you wouldn't normally do. Give yourself a manicure and pedicure, soak in a hot bubble bath, get a massage, engage in some retail therapy (shopping!), go to dinner with a friend, or have a movie marathon with all your favorites.

Attend a support group

Though you may not think you have time for a support group now, it is more important than ever to attend. These groups can help you feel less alone and support you in any struggles you may be having. Just make sure you call ahead to find out whether the particular group you're interested in is what will meet your needs.

Keep in touch

Find a friend or family member whom you trust to talk to and share your feelings and frustrations with.

Try counseling

Unfortunately, many caregivers don't take time for counseling until their caregiving gig is over, but it's a good idea to talk with a counselor while in the midst of caregiving. Professional counseling can help you deal with difficult emotions, including anger, anxiety, grief, and guilt. This may be especially important if you're caring for someone who has both Parkinson's and dementia, as that can be extra trying on you.

Get regular checkups

Visit your doctor regularly to get your health checked. Whether it be a mammogram, prostate test, colon cancer test, or flu or pneumonia vaccination, you must schedule time for medical tests and checkups. Think of it as preventative maintenance for your caregiving machine. After all, if your health declines, you won't be able to care for your loved one.

If you and your doctor agree that you need to take medications because of stress, you can use them in conjunction with the strategies discussed here.

Exercise

It is a well-known fact that exercise is not only good for your physical health but also a great way to reduce stress and anxiety and relieve depression. Exercise is important for both the caregiver and the person with PD. If it works for both of you, you may choose to attend an exercise, yoga, or tai chi class together at a local community or fitness center.

Other exercises you may want to choose are walking (outside or on a treadmill), swimming, dancing, or lifting weights (appropriate for your level of fitness). Whatever you choose, make sure it's something you like to do and keep moving!

Laugh a little

Try to maintain a sense of humor while caregiving. This may sound very simple, but one of the biggest ways you can reduce stress is through laughter. Yes, laughter really can be the best medicine. Recent studies suggest that laughter can help in many ways to heal the mind and body.[14]

Laughter therapy clubs are emerging across the U.S. and Canada. If you think this sounds crazy or that it couldn't work, check out World Laughter Tour's website at https://www.worldlaughtertour .com/. For a slight twist on the laughter club, there are also laughter yoga clubs all over the world. You can find one near you by visiting Laughter Yoga's website at https://laughteryoga.org/finder /find-club/.

Try pet therapy

If you have a pet, you probably don't need convincing that animals can have a positive effect on your mood and overall health. Holding or playing with your dog or cat can provide much-needed comfort and laughs.

If you don't have a pet, try spending time with one. Even something as simple as watching the fish in an aquarium or a goldfish pond can be very relaxing.

Get help!

As I mention throughout this book many times, don't forget to ask for help from family, friends, support groups, and your local Parkinson's foundation. Let them know if you're feeling burned out by caregiver stress. You'll be surprised at who comes out of the woodwork when you let people know you need help.

12. Keeping Your Cool: How to Stay Patient During Those Trying Times

"The one sure thing that my family has learned is patience. My mom has to be a little bit slower and take her time at most tasks. Instead of feeling like I need to rush her, I take the time to help her any way that I can and treasure every moment that I can spend with her." —KATHY V., PARKINSON'S CAREGIVER

Anger isn't an emotion I'm overly comfortable with; I usually try to avoid it if I can. Sure, if you push my buttons over and over or offend my deepest convictions, I will stand up for myself, but in general I try to steer clear of volatile situations.

When it comes to caregiving, I have to admit there were a few moments when I lost my patience and was not as coolheaded as I'd like to have been with my mom.

Here's some comforting news: all caregivers lose it sometimes. We lose patience, we yell, we have meltdowns. The important thing is what we do with that anger.

There are several things you can do to help manage difficult emotions.

- Remind yourself that you're angry and frustrated with the situation, *not* your loved one.
- Don't beat yourself up for it—forgive yourself and move on.
- Acknowledge that you're exhausted and emotional. Know that it's common for caregivers to snap at their loved ones once in a while, especially when in this state.
- Take slow, deep breaths to get control over your body—then you'll have a better chance of gaining control of your emotions. Sounds simple, but it works!

- As always, reach out for help! Getting help to ease your caregiver load can give you much-needed rest and help prevent potential anger episodes.
- Find ways to let off steam. Exercise, write in a journal, go out with a friend, or just plain ol' scream (somewhere private, of course!).
- If you find yourself getting angry frequently, talk to a counselor, therapist, or clergyperson to help you find ways to manage that.

13. How to Deal With Guilt

"I feel guilty for not doing everything for my husband (who has advanced PD). I know I'm doing my best to take care of him, but sometimes it doesn't feel like enough."

—SANDRA W., PARKINSON'S CAREGIVER

I wish someone had taught me early on in my caregiving journey about guilt. I wrestled with this emotion for a very long time, not knowing what to do with it or how common it was.

Here's a news flash about caregiving: you're going to feel guilty a lot of the time. Guilty for not doing enough. Guilty for not being there enough. Guilty for losing your temper, making wrong decisions, or breaking promises. Guilt was such a part of my life that I felt guilty every time I was having fun and my mom wasn't.

Here are some key points and strategies to help you deal with guilt.

- Remind yourself that experiencing guilt is *normal.*
- Acknowledge that you're doing your best.
- Realize that no matter how much time you spend with your loved one trying to meet all their needs, guilt will make you feel like it's never enough. Guilt can eat you alive. Don't let it.
- Try a mantra (e.g., "I love my mom and I'm doing the best I can").
- Don't fall into the "I shoulda or coulda" trap. Things are what they are and stewing about it just wastes time and energy.
- Know that there are two types of guilt: good guilt and bad guilt. Good guilt can help you make positive changes by pointing out little things to improve in your behavior. For example, if you feel guilty because you were impatient with your loved one, good guilt will remind you to try to be a bit

more patient next time. Bad guilt, on the other hand, does nothing for you except make you feel bad about a situation you can't control, or one that is actually good for you (e.g., hiring home care because you can't do it all yourself).

- Instead of focusing on the things you're not doing right for your loved one, focus on the things you are doing right.

14. How to Cope With Loneliness

"I feel strongly that emotional well-being is a huge part of this and since a lot of people with Parkinson's also suffer from anxiety, anxiety management and information on relaxation techniques should be standard medical practice."

—ANONYMOUS, PARKINSON'S CAREGIVER

Caregiving can be a lonely job. It can isolate you from friends because they can't relate to your demanding life. It can make you feel so tired or depressed that going out feels like too much work, so instead you stay at home feeling lonely.

If you're experiencing feelings of loneliness, know that many other caregivers out there are feeling the same. With just a bit of effort, you can help lessen this feeling by keeping connected with the right friends and/or family members. Though some friendships may fade, your close friends will stand by you if you can help them help you. Here are some ways you can do this.

- Understand your friends' limits. Not everyone will be able or willing to take the long caregiver journey with you—it's tough.
- Give direction. Sometimes friends want to help but don't know how. They may also find it hard to relate to you now. If this is the case, talk to them and let them know what you need; that sometimes all you want is for them to be there and listen.
- Hang on to your friends and let them know how much you appreciate them.
- Get out once in a while! Though you may not feel like socializing, just being around others can keep depression at bay. Go to the movies, go out for lunch, or go on a walk with one or more friends. Force yourself to take a break from caregiving at least once a week!

15. How to Handle Depression

"My best advice to all who have this disease is to carry on. The thing I find that helps a lot is when my mate takes me around to the club for a beer or two. I see my mates and after two hours all I can say is that a laugh and a smile are far better than medication. This is what I find helps in my life." —JIM, PWP

While I was battling depression in my teens, I remember my mom telling me that she couldn't be happy until I was better. "A mother is only as happy as her unhappiest child," she'd say. In caring for my mom, I came to understand what she meant by that.

Caring for someone with Parkinson's has its share of challenges, and one of the biggest is dealing with the depression that can accompany it. If you're not diligent, your loved one's depression can cause you to get depressed as well, so learning about this side of Parkinson's is very important for both of you.

Depression is very common in people with Parkinson's. It's not unusual for someone to feel sad and possibly get depressed after being diagnosed with a chronic illness like PD. It's also important to know that depression is a clinical symptom of the disease as well. In fact, up to 50 percent of people with Parkinson's may suffer from some form of depression during the course of their disease.[15]

If your loved one suffers from depression, it will most definitely affect you, too. Because depression is the number one issue that prevents people from living a happy and full life, it is extremely important that you be on the lookout for signs of depression in your loved one. Depression can also increase the physical effects of PD and may cause a progression of the disease.

If you observe your loved one experiencing five or more of the following symptoms for longer than two weeks at a time, you should contact their doctor.

- Unhappy mood
- Inability to enjoy things they once enjoyed
- Changes in appetite
- Sleeping problems (either oversleeping or inability to sleep)
- Excessive tiredness
- Change in level of activity
- Concentration problems
- Low self-esteem
- Talking about death

Fortunately, for most people with Parkinson's, depression can be controlled. Treatment for depression typically yields the best results when patients receive both psychological therapy and the proper medication for their symptoms. Psychological therapy can help people with Parkinson's regain their sense of self-worth, cope with stress, and maintain positive relationships with the people around them, including caregivers and family members.

There are many antidepressant medications available, each with its own advantages and disadvantages. Most people with PD should not take Asendin (amoxapine) because this medication could temporarily worsen PD symptoms. Your loved one's doctor will know which medications are best for them.

* * *

Here's a little story to finish this topic of depression. You may wish to share this with your loved one if they need a little encouragement. When my mom was first diagnosed, a family member suggested she go to a support group for people with Parkinson's. When she arrived, she encountered a room full of sad-looking people in wheelchairs. This was very discouraging and depressing for her, as she barely had any noticeable symptoms of PD at this point.

In that moment she made a crucial decision. She decided that as much as possible, she wasn't going to let Parkinson's bring her down. She also decided that she was going to do all she could to keep her independence for as long as possible. "Don't let anyone take away your independence," Mom used to say. In other words, don't give up and say, "Oh well, I have Parkinson's. I guess I'm doomed to X, Y, or Z."

Mom made it over 15 years with Parkinson's before she relied on a wheelchair for any length of time. Now, we all know that every case of Parkinson's is different, and maybe my mom got "the good kind," but I believe that it was also her strong will, determination, faith, and positive outlook that helped her live for 30 years with this disease.

Make sure you check with the pharmacist about any new medications (like antidepressants) because some may not be compatible with your loved one's PD medications.

16. How to Cope With Worries About the Unknown

"We try not to be naive, keep informed with all the latest information, and laugh A LOT while planning realistically for what might be. It's a fine balance."

—ANONYMOUS, PARKINSON'S CAREGIVER

I always thought my mom to be a bit of a worrywart, which is probably where I got my worrying tendencies. It's not like I don't know it's bad for me—I know it is—but facing giants like Parkinson's and dementia made me more worried about the future than ever before. Intellectually I know that no one can predict or control what lies ahead, but throughout Mom's illness, I found it hard not to worry about how it would eventually all end. Would she suffer? Also, would I develop PD years down the road?

If there's one thing in life I used to think was controllable, it was one's health. Just eat right, exercise regularly, and avoid stress and you'll make it till at least your 70s with no major health issues. But when Mom was diagnosed with Parkinson's in her late 40s and my sister with cancer in her mid-40s, I had to face the fact that maybe we can't entirely control our health.

Over the past little while, I've been working on eliminating my fears of future ill health and other unknowns. I now know that fear of the unknown is nothing more than a mental obstacle, one that has been getting in the way of my being able to live my life to the fullest.

If you're caring for a loved one with Parkinson's, you may be worried about their future as well. I know it can be scary, not having control over their fate. Unfortunately it's impossible to predict the course of this disease, so it's best to work on controlling the things you can and avoid worrying about the things you can't.

If you've been burdened with fear and worry about the unknown, you'll be happy to know that you can get rid of these by applying some of the following strategies in your life.

Fight your fear

To best fight your fear, you need to understand the cause of it. Fear is a natural human instinct and almost all of us fear something in our lives. Fear of the unknown stems from certain things, situations, or memories in life.

Ask yourself, "What do I fear the most? What situations do I frequently avoid in my day-to-day life?" Once you figure out the root cause of your fear, you'll find it easier to beat it.

Educate yourself

Sometimes fear of the unknown is based on factors that are beyond our control. In these cases, educating yourself about the fear and learning about the actual risk is the best way to ease your fear.

For instance, if you fear being diagnosed with Parkinson's down the road, learning about the stats on who gets PD and what the risk factors are may help you. I sometimes go down the road of, "If I get Parkinson's, who will take care of me? How will I pay for all my medical costs? Will I end up with dementia in the end?" These are all legit questions, and the first two I can somewhat plan for if I choose to, which helps ease my fear. I can't control whether or not I get dementia, though, so worrying about that is just wasted time and energy.

Mom used to fear that she'd get trapped in the house in a fire or tornado when she was immobile and nobody would be there to help her out. This fear may appear dramatic, but I understood the helplessness she felt when her PD made her stuck in place, so I assured her over and over again that someone would be there to help her in an emergency.

Our minds tend to dwell on worst-case scenarios, but the worst may not happen at all. Michael J. Fox once said, "If you imagine the worst-case scenario, and it comes true, you've lived it twice." I try to remind myself that worrying doesn't do anything other than make me more stressed and susceptible to illness.

Confront your fear!

Often we tend to run from situations that induce fear; in the process, we may lose certain opportunities in life. If you want to experience all that life has to offer, you must move out of your comfort zone and confront your fears.

One way to confront your fear is to take action. For example, if you fear an uncertain financial future, talking with a financial or estate planner may help.

Practice visualization meditation

Visualization meditation will help you focus on the positives rather than on your fear. To do this, find a quiet place away from any noise so that you can meditate peacefully. Once seated in your quiet place, visualize in your mind how you are going to fight your fear, step-by-step. Imagine yourself conquering your fear every day. Winning the battle in your mind will help you take real action.

Take baby steps

If you're living with a fear that can cause no real harm to you, take baby steps to eliminate it. For instance, if you have a fear of public speaking, speak in front of a small group of friends or family. Taking baby steps will allow you to conquer your fear over a period of time.

Fight fear with fun!

Don't take your life too seriously. Once the time is gone, you can't get it back. Wasting too much time being worried or fearful of the unknown is just that—a waste.

16. How to Cope With Worries About the Unknown

Humor is a great way to rid yourself of the fear of the unknown. Do something fun with friends or watch a funny movie—anything to get rid of those unwanted thoughts in your head.

A common fear for Parkinson's caregivers is how their loved one will ultimately pass. I worried about my mom a lot, hoping she wouldn't choke to death (choking can become an issue later on in PD as swallowing becomes more difficult) or suffer a long, painful ending. To combat this, I kept my focus on the things I could control (e.g., making sure all her foods were easy to swallow) and not on the things I couldn't. I also focused on my faith and hers as well. In the end, Mom passed away quietly in her sleep after a brief bout of pneumonia. I was comforted in knowing that she was now in heaven.

17. How to Deal With Resentment

"I am sitting here trying to understand how to deal with the loneliness and resentment I feel for giving up my own home and life. I have been sleeping on the floor at my parents' for the last two years and have given up all but my job to care for them. Don't get me wrong, I love my parents to death, but I have been caring for my dad (who has Parkinson's) for about ten years now. It started out slowly but now is a full-time job."

—ANONYMOUS, PARKINSON'S CAREGIVER

The above sentiment, shared with me by a fellow Parkinson's caregiver, is one felt by many caregivers. Whether directed toward Parkinson's, the situation in general, or your loved one, it's tough for even the most willing caregivers to fend off resentment all of the time.

Resentment is a very human emotion, so don't beat yourself up if you feel it toward the person you're caring for. Almost all caregivers feel this way at one time or another. After all, it's hard to accept that the life you planned and hoped to have with your loved one isn't going to come to fruition.

Here are a few tips to help you deal with resentment.

- Remind yourself that, above all, it's the situation you're resentful of. It's rarely the person in your care who's causing your feelings; what you're upset about is almost always the disease, the burden of caregiving, and the changes to all your lives. Try not to feel guilty for feeling this way.
- As hard as it may be at first, try to let go of some of the past and future. If you dwell on what might have been, you'll find resentment creeping in. Instead, focus on being in the present and look for the good things in the life you share with your loved one.

- Find an outlet for resentment so that it doesn't consume you. Be it exercising, talking with a friend, writing in a journal, or even screaming it out (somewhere private), it is important that you have healthy ways to vent your feelings.
- Don't let caregiving be the only thing in your life. Make time to do things that make you happy—this will make you a better caregiver in the end.

PART 4

Getting Practical:
General Caregiving Issues

18. How to Help When Help Isn't Wanted

"My husband had a very difficult time accepting the fact that he has Parkinson's. It took a lot of patience, love, and caring to help him along. Most importantly, I learned that no matter what I did or said or tried to do to help him in every way, he still had to experience every stage of acceptance on his own."

—ANONYMOUS, PARKINSON'S CAREGIVER

It's tough to watch your loved one go through the challenges that come with Parkinson's. Progressively losing mobility is just one of the many losses they have to deal with, and each one brings with it a sense that they are slowly losing their independence and freedom. These losses can also deal a significant blow to their self-esteem.

Many aging adults refuse help from their younger family members because it reminds them of their age. Even though family members mean well, they sometimes offer help in a way that challenges their older loved one's identity as an independent adult.

The thing is, most older adults don't need or want to be reminded that they are old. In fact, one study found that this is the main reason they refuse help.[16] When their identities are threatened, older people may even lash out, sometimes in a dangerous manner, to prove their youth.

As a caregiver for someone with Parkinson's, you'll want to keep your loved one safe while they get the care and help they need. The challenge will be to do this without overstepping your boundaries, causing them to become resentful and resist your help.

Here are a few ways to help your loved one when they're resistant to your help.

Ask, don't order

If your loved one believes that asking for help was their idea, they may be more likely to accept your help. If you start by lending a hand with just those things for which your loved one admits to needing help, they may be more receptive to any future suggestions you have regarding their need for outside assistance.

Often you may find the person you are caring for getting frustrated because they are unable to complete certain daily activities that they once were able to. One common area of frustration is walking. Depending on their stage of Parkinson's, you may be able to help a person with PD overcome some of their difficulties.

For example, my mom frequently had trouble walking when her meds started to wear off. Often when that happened, she would get frustrated and forget that she knew other ways of getting from point A to point B. Here's where the caregiver can jump in and offer some suggestions to help out. In Mom's case we would make a suggestion: "Why don't you try walking sideways?" She would do it and then immediately be on her way.

We didn't need to be telling Mom what to do. We would simply suggest—or ask her if she'd like to try—another method of walking. That way she was still choosing what she would like to do and didn't feel ordered around.

R-E-S-P-E-C-T

Remember to show respect in everything you do with your loved one, as it is the foundation upon which all good relationships are built. One way to do that is to ask them for permission before you rush in to help them with something. For example, before you assume that it's okay for you to sit in on their doctor appointments, ask them how they feel about that. If your loved one prefers, one option is to remain in the waiting room and arrange to speak with the doctor after the appointment is over.

Ask to help with little things first

Even if your loved one doesn't want your help with a specific task, they may allow you to help them if you ask to help out a little. Just make sure that when you do lend them a hand, you don't end up taking over. Remember, the goal is to help them keep their independence, sense of purpose, and self-worth.

If your loved one needs help with their daily activities, you may suggest a home support worker or someone who can help them out from time to time (like another family member or a friend). Sometimes people accept help from "outsiders" more readily than they do from their close family members.

Also, you could suggest that the support worker (or whomever) come out on a trial basis. That way, your loved can see the benefits of having outside help.

> Always remember that safety should come first. If you have to assume total control of a task to make sure that your loved one is safe, do it.

19. What NOT to Do When Caregiving

"Put aside part of each day for conversation, as opposed to watching TV or merely dishing out pills and food. Make sure that the conversation involves listening and is two-way."

—CAMILLA O., PARKINSON'S CAREGIVER

Caregiving is a process of trial and error. You will make mistakes from time to time, but learning from them is the key. There are a few things you'll want to avoid doing that will help you out in your caregiving journey.

Following are a few of the don'ts in caregiving.

Don't try to fix everything at once

You've probably been told this before, but it's worth repeating: pick your battles. Your loved one may need help with many tasks and you may discover that they want things done in a way that is different from the way you'd do them. Remember that your goal should be to help them, not fix them. Prioritize their needs and work with them to tackle one task at a time.

Don't patronize

Sometimes, as an aging loved one becomes more fragile, we start treating them more like children than adults. Don't do this. Even if you're caring for someone with dementia, be careful not to talk down to them. Treat your loved one the way you'd want to be treated.

Don't interrupt

Make sure you're really listening to what your loved one is saying. Try not to interrupt or be tempted to talk when there is silence during a conversation. When it's your turn to speak, reflect to your loved one what they said and then ask them if you got it right.

Don't advise unless it's asked for

An especially important tip for adult children who are looking after their aging parents is to not give unsolicited advice. Your mother and father are used to providing you with advice and guidance, so when this dynamic begins to shift, they may lose their self-esteem and feel out of control. Hiring an outside expert (such as a financial advisor or an elder law attorney) to provide professional guidance can make an elder more receptive to new information.

Don't forget about how they feel

It's always a good idea to think about others before yourself. If you put yourself in your loved one's shoes, you will come to understand that they feel that their independence and freedom are being threatened. Always show empathy and sensitivity.

Don't argue

One thing I learned very early on in my caregiving journey is that I am not my mother. She had different ways of seeing things and doing things, and because of this we didn't always see eye to eye. Remember to acknowledge your loved one's questions, concerns, and viewpoints. Compromising was something I learned to do to reduce the number of our disagreements.

Don't forget about your tone

Though your patience will be tested throughout your caregiving journey, it's important that you pay attention to your tone when you're talking with your loved one. Speak calmly and avoid raising your voice or being condescending, both of which can quickly turn a conversation into an argument that can then escalate into something even bigger.

If your loved one has difficulty hearing, make sure to enunciate your words so they can really hear what you're saying. Nothing's worse than having an argument start over something you didn't even say!

20. Long-Distance Caregiving

"I remind myself that it's okay to make mistakes in caring for my mom; after all, we are learning about this disease together. I rely on my faith to help me through the tough times."

—ANONYMOUS, PARKINSON'S CAREGIVER

For a few years during Mom's illness, I cared for her while living 2,500 miles away. I won't lie—it was tough. When I lived nearby, it was a lot easier to know how she was doing and what her needs were. Though I tried my best to keep up-to-date with her health and to help her via telephone, sometimes it felt like it wasn't enough.

I went through all kinds of emotions, including guilt over not being able to visit more often, frustration over not being able to help as much as I once could, and worry over the level of care she was receiving. I struggled with letting go and depending on others to care for her.

If you're a long-distance caregiver you can probably relate to some of this. Maybe you spend your long weekends or vacations visiting your loved one, hoping and praying that each time you visit they'll still be okay. You're not alone. A recent study found that up to one-third of all caregivers care for their loved ones from a distance, and most struggle with the things I just mentioned.[17]

Though there will be challenges along the way, following are some things you can do to make caring for your loved one from a distance easier.

Communicate

Communication is crucial in caregiving. Communicating with those who are involved with caring for your loved one locally can help you keep on top of their changing needs. This will help you know if or when they need more skilled help in their home or, if they're in a care facility, what changes in care, medications, diet, and so forth need to be made to their daily regimen.

So, what can long-distance relatives do to be helpful, short of moving back home? Let your loved one and the primary caregiver know that you are still there for them.

Get local help

If you find that you can't keep track of all that is needed for your loved one from afar, there's a relatively new service that may be able to help you. Consider hiring a geriatric care manager (also known as aging life care) who can be your liaison and provide services, including arranging financial, legal, and medical services and assisting with a move from home to a care facility.

It is important to note that not all geriatric care managers are required to be certified by their state or the federal government, so make sure that you interview them yourself and/or do a thorough check with their organization before you hire them.

Be kind to yourself

Long-distance caregiving can be emotionally draining. If you're like me, you'll probably experience a range of emotions. Getting a support system in place is really important to help you handle your emotions. Sometimes after a Skype call with my mom, I just needed a hug. Thankfully, my very supportive husband was always there to give me one (or more!).

Connect with family

If your family doesn't get together very often, you may find that when you do, your talks tend to center on the subject of Parkinson's and your loved one's care needs. Though this may be necessary, sometimes we need to be reminded to take a break from that and talk about other things. A good heart-to-heart talk with my sister is something we both benefit from.

Set up weekly phone or video call dates

I always looked forward to Mondays and Thursdays at 5 p.m. That's when I got to Skype (video call) my mom to see how she was doing and tell her my swimming stories. If you ask me, video calling is one of the greatest communication inventions in recent times. It made such a positive difference for my mom and me while I was her long-distance caregiver.

Many parents with adult children think that they are bothering them by calling, so they don't. Another reason they don't call is that they believe, as my mom used to say, "it costs a fortune." Even though she's wrong (most video calls are free or virtually free), I made it easier on her by being the one who picked up the phone.

Setting up a regular Skype (or phone) date with your loved one is not only a great way to see how they're doing and get a chance to share your life with them, it also gives your loved one something to look forward to regularly, which can mean a lot.

Get peace of mind

The best way to find peace of mind in caregiving is knowing that your loved one is safe and that their care needs are being met. Obtaining this information and staying in the loop can be hard when you live far away. Often you get second-hand details on your loved one, making it hard to know exactly what's going on.

To remedy this, you want to get as many eyes on the situation as you can. Connect with those who interact with your loved one, whether it be your loved one's primary caregiver at home or nurses and support workers at a care facility where they live. If they go for a doctor's appointment, call afterward and ask how it went.

Take the time to find professionals who can help your loved one. If need be, hire an elder law attorney to make sure your loved one's finances and insurance needs are taken care of.

Plan for the future

Planning for an emergency isn't exactly fun, but it can be helpful. Of course, you can't plan for every possible scenario, but knowing what you might do if your loved one has a fall or if their condition worsens can help you face and deal with the situation more easily if it does happen.

I have to admit that my family didn't plan for when my mom first had a bad fall and had to be rushed to the emergency room to get 16 stitches in her head. It was scary, but thankfully my sister and I were close by and were able to be with and comfort my mom while she was in the hospital.

Educate yourself

If you're not already versed in All Things Parkinson's, you should at least have a basic understanding of the disease. This will help you support your loved one and anyone who may be caring for them close by. You can start by Googling your national Parkinson's foundation or going to AllAboutParkinsons.com. There you can find information on diagnosis, symptoms, treatment options, nutrition and exercise regimens, and a whole lot more.

Make sure you know your loved one's current needs and the medications they're taking. Keep a contact list of their doctor, neurologist, pharmacist, and any health care workers who are involved in caring for your loved one. You may also want to have financial and legal documents available in case they're needed.

Check in on finances

Talking about money is always tricky, so be sure that when you do speak to your loved one about this topic, you do so tactfully. Many people won't ask for financial help even if they're in dire straits, but if there's a need and you can help, offer to do so. If your loved one won't accept monetary assistance, they may take your help in purchasing needed items for their care or allow you to help pay for utility bills, transportation costs, or housecleaning or yard services.

Be kind to your loved one's caregivers

Let those who are caring for your loved one close by know that they are appreciated. Whether it be something as simple as a thank you card, flowers, or something more elaborate like a gift basket, such shows of appreciation can mean a lot to someone who may be tired from all the demands of caregiving.

Visit when you can

Decide how many times a month or year you can afford to visit and budget for it. When you do visit, try to do so when your loved one has an appointment with the neurologist so that you can be there for it. This can be beneficial for both you and the doctor.

Also, when you're visiting, don't add to the primary caregiver's stress level by asking or expecting them to put you up or take care of you.

Know that all visits are important

If your loved one has developed dementia along with their Parkinson's, it's likely that they do not connect with you the way they used to when you visit. Many long-distance caregivers find this very painful and wonder if their visits are still valuable.

I experienced this while visiting my mom in the nursing home. A few times she'd been so agitated that I questioned whether my being there was making her life better or worse. That's when I reminded myself that I wasn't there just to visit. I used some of my time to talk with the nurses, personal support workers, and volunteers who were all part of Mom's care team. This helped me get a better idea of how she was doing on a day-to-day basis and in what ways I could help her. Something as simple as finding out that she needed long socks (her short ones kept falling off during episodes of dyskinesia) made me feel better, as it gave me something specific that I could do to help her.

I also was able to speak to her doctor, who agreed to make a medication change (I had discovered that Mom was being given unnecessary pain meds for a fall months earlier), and to her physical therapist about making changes to her wheelchair to make it more comfortable for her.

Help the primary caregiver

Living far away may mean that you can't personally cover for your loved one's primary caregiver, but you can offer to pay for respite care. This could be at an extended care facility or at your home if your loved one is able to travel.

If and when the time comes, don't shy away from agreeing to a decision to have your loved one moved to a residential care facility. Respect the fact that you're not the one providing the day-to-day care and that you don't know how much of a burden the primary caregiver has.

Try not to let finances or egos get in the way of doing what's best for those whose lives are most affected.

Long-distance caregiving NOs

As a long-distance caregiver, you have ways to support your loved one's primary caregiver. Following are a few points to remember.

- Don't underestimate anything. Being away from your loved one may make you susceptible to underestimating the severity of their day-to-day symptoms and what level of caregiver burden they can be. Providing physical care, particularly for someone with advanced Parkinson's, can be physically demanding, so be sensitive to the primary caregiver's needs.
- Be careful about offering advice. Because you aren't with your loved one on a day-to-day basis, you may not have an accurate reading of how things are going with them. If you have points of wisdom you'd like to offer your loved one's primary caregiver, do so carefully and avoid criticizing them.
- Don't make promises you can't keep. Though you may mean well, it's important that you don't make promises to your loved one that you may not be able to keep. Instead of saying things like, "Don't worry, Mom, we'd never put you in a home," be empathetic and tell your loved one that you will talk about other options if and when the time comes.

21. What to Do When No One Will Help

"Remember to laugh together. Maintain a sense of humor about the situations you find yourselves in. If there is anything you had wanted to do as a couple, do it before it's too late; a cruise, a vacation of any type—do it even if you have to borrow the money. The memories are a wonderful balm to the loneliness."

—SHARRON H., PARKINSON'S CAREGIVER

Caregiving is tough, and even more so when other family members won't help and you feel that you have to do it all on your own. It's not uncommon for there to be one person in the family who has to step up and take on most of the burden of caregiving. If this has happened to you, you know how it can make you feel: resentful, stressed out, and overwhelmed.

So why does this happen? Everyone copes with Parkinson's in different ways. Some family members may go into denial, some may get depressed, and others may make themselves busy trying to do everything. You may look at a family member and think that they aren't helping, but it could just be their way of dealing with a particular problem. This is why talking to your family is so important. Many conflicts can be avoided through simple communication. This doesn't necessarily mean that your family members will help out, but at least by talking with them you can get a better understanding of where they're coming from.

Here are a few things to keep in mind when no one will help.

- Understand that everyone reacts and copes in different ways.
- Before you give up on receiving help from family members, make sure you have asked them directly for help.

Sometimes caregivers complain about siblings not helping when they actually haven't given them a chance to.

- Make a care plan that can be changed as needed.
- Get respite care to prevent burnout! Find out what resources and services are available in the area (things like transportation, meal delivery, companionship, etc.).
- If family won't help, find alternate sources. Don't waste energy being angry and frustrated about it. It's not worth it.
- Keep asking for help until you get the kind and amount you need. DON'T GIVE UP!

PART 5

Getting Practical: Caregiving For Parkinson's

22. Caregiving in the Early Stages of PD

"I think it is very important to look for the positive and smile and really laugh a lot. It is commonly believed in the medical field that good belly laughs are good for your health. I have friends who email me every day with funny stories, etc., and I look for funny shows on TV." —WILMA S., PWP

As you begin the journey of Parkinson's with your loved one, you'll probably have a lot of questions. You'll also most likely have a lot of new information and advice thrown at you that you'll have to sift through.

Because Parkinson's affects everyone differently, no caregiving journey will be the same. As a caregiver for someone with Parkinson's, you have to learn and adapt as you go. Just remember that your journey will be a team effort and you don't have to—and shouldn't—go it alone!

Here are some suggestions to help you care for your loved one in the early stages of Parkinson's.

Educate yourself

When you are first starting out as a Parkinson's caregiver, you'll want to learn the basics of the disease—things like identifying the various stages, learning and managing symptoms, and understanding medications and their side effects. There are many resources available for caregivers, but the best place to start is your national Parkinson's foundation or society. You can find them online, and they can also direct you to your local chapter, where you can find out about any support groups that may be in your area.

Learning about Parkinson's is just one aspect of educating yourself, as you'll want to learn about the specific ways in which the disease is affecting your loved one as well. As you care for them, observe them closely to detect any changes in their motor function (ability to move) and mood.

Because your loved one might not be aware of their changing abilities, you can be their extra set of eyes. This will enable you to give them better emotional and physical support.

As mentioned earlier, caring for someone with Parkinson's requires learning and adapting as you go. The more you can learn about Parkinson's during the early stages, the more you will be able to take part in health care discussions and make informed decisions in the future.

Learn to adapt

When you first hear that your loved one has Parkinson's, it can come as a real shock. Your life may seem like it has been turned entirely upside down, and you may feel unqualified for taking on the caregiving role. Feeling this way is common; however, caregiver is a role you can learn and grow into.

You may have many questions, including whether you should get a second opinion, how you will share the diagnosis with the family, and how you will balance your needs with those of your loved one. These are all good questions to ask.

In many cases, getting a second opinion is a good idea, as long as it's from someone who's qualified—like a neurologist who specializes in Parkinson's. When it comes to sharing the diagnosis with family and friends, talk with your loved one about how they want to do this. If you have children living at home, make sure you tell them in an age-appropriate way.

Because Parkinson's is a progressive disease, your loved one's needs will change. As they do, so will your caregiving responsibilities. Communicate with your loved one about your needs as well to make sure that you are taking care of yourself throughout your caregiving journey.

Be patient

One very important habit you'll need to learn or develop as a caregiver for someone with Parkinson's is patience. I can't tell you how many times I've heard from Parkinson's caregivers that the number one thing you need to learn is to be patient with your loved one!

Some days your loved one's symptoms will be pronounced, while other days not as much. Ask if you can help your loved one with tasks, but don't assume that they want help because they may not. Be patient and allow them to do things on their own, even if it takes longer. Trying to rush your loved one will only get them frustrated and stressed and slow them down even more.

It takes time to learn everything there is to know about caring for someone with Parkinson's, so don't forget to be patient with yourself as well.

Provide reassurance

Reassuring your loved one, especially in the early stages after diagnosis, can really help. Remind them that Parkinson's disease progresses slowly in most people and that they can still live a full life.

Because depression is so prevalent in people with Parkinson's, it never hurts to offer a hug or two, or any kind of physical touch. Let your loved one know you're in this together.

Talk to someone who's been there

It may be helpful for you and your loved one to talk to an experienced caregiver—one who has "been there, done that" and can share strategies on how to deal with the various situations you may face. That person may also be able to reassure you that Parkinson's is a slowly progressing disease for most people and that it can be lived with—and lived with well.

Try a support group

Attending a support group can be a good way to educate yourself about Parkinson's and also learn new ways to care for your loved one.

Find out whether there's a Parkinson's or Parkinson's caregiver support group in your area by checking your local newspaper for community announcements of meetings, or look online for your local Parkinson's chapter, which will be able to tell you about any support groups that may be in your area.

If you are unable to locate a support group specifically for Parkinson's caregivers, there may be general caregiving support groups in your area that could be beneficial. Remember, many of the issues you face are universal to all caregivers. Make sure you call the group's moderator ahead of time to ensure that the group will be the right fit for you.

23. Caregiving in the Mid-Stages of PD

"I bought a battery-operated doorbell and put the base unit in the central part of the house. I then velcroed the buzzer part to my husband's wheelchair. I also attached a piece of Velcro to the nightstand by his bed. That way we could attach the doorbell there when he was in bed. This had a pleasant chime sound and was very helpful in him letting me know he needed me."

—SHARRON H., PARKINSON'S CAREGIVER

Caring for someone with Parkinson's can be both rewarding and challenging. Because Parkinson's progresses at different rates for different people, it is impossible to predict what changes you will face and when you will face them. However, there are things you can do to prepare yourself as a caregiver for the changes that are likely to occur.

Get into a routine

Scheduling is essential, especially when it comes to medications and meals. Because some Parkinson's meds must be taken at specific times before and after meals, it's helpful to establish a medication and meal schedule so that it becomes routine.

Plan

As mentioned in chapter 9 on planning, there are several legal documents that you should have drawn up to make sure your loved one gets the kind of care they want in the later stages. These include a HIPAA authorization, a health care and financial power of attorney, a living will or advanced care directive, a will, and a trust.

In terms of day-to-day planning, allow extra time for things. For example, when we used to get ready to go shopping with Mom, it would take 15 minutes, but as her disease progressed, that would sometimes increase to 30 minutes or more.

Speaking of planning, if your loved one is no longer able to drive, you may want to help them plan alternative means of transportation. There are several options out there, including public transit, ride-sharing, and community shuttle services.

One thing concerning planning for mealtimes, especially if your loved one has trouble chewing or swallowing, is that you may want to learn the Heimlich maneuver. This is used to dislodge food stuck in the throat if the person is choking and could be a lifesaver.

Another thing to consider in the mid-stages of PD is to plan around your loved one's on and off times. If you know your loved one's mobility is generally best at certain times of day, plan outings then. For example, Mom's mobility was at its worst in the morning when she first got up. That was largely due to the timing of her medications, but also because her body hadn't been moving for six to eight hours (and we all know how hard it is to get a non-PD body going in the morning sometimes!).

Knowing when her worst times of day for mobility were helped us plan appointments accordingly. For example, doctor and physio appointments were better in the early afternoon. If we had a shopping day planned (Mom *loved* to shop), we scheduled in breaks for meds and always made sure we had walker or wheelchair available if she were to lose her "wheels."

Keep in mind that although planning around on/off times is ideal, it's not always possible as these cycles can be unpredictable.

Get in tune with medications

As Parkinson's progresses, you will notice inconsistencies in how your loved one reacts to medications. For example, on some days they'll have lots of mobility and on others not. These on/off fluctuations in response to the medication levodopa are common.

As we know, the goal of PD drug therapy is to increase on times and decrease off times. As a caregiver, it's important to know that though it takes on average 20 to 30 minutes for levodopa to kick in, this varies from person to person and can be very unpredictable. How long the on time lasts varies as well. It can depend on everything from how long your loved one has had the disease to what they've had to eat.

As a sidebar, the dosage of medication neurologists prescribe is usually based on an educated guess. What they do, especially over time, is to overshoot by giving the patient more than they need. This can give your loved one the side effect of dyskinesia (the uncontrolled movements you may have seen in someone with PD). It can be tricky to find the balance between getting the most on time without too much dyskinesia.

Mom experienced dyskinesia a lot, especially in the mid to late stages of the disease, and it was a real pain in the butt. At times it would get in the way of her being able to eat. Also, she moved so much because of it that we figured she was burning double the calories she normally would have.

We worked hard at controlling the dyskinesia. Mom took a med to help ease it (amantadine), which had its own side effect of hallucinations. If this happens to your loved one, you will have to work closely with their neurologist to find the best solution.

Think about safety concerns

If your loved one's symptoms start to affect their mobility, memory, or thinking skills significantly, you may have to consider whether it is safe for them to perform certain daily activities. For example, driving a car may be dangerous for them, your family, and others on the road. However, giving up driving can be very hard for some people, and it increases the burden on the caregiver. (You can read more about making decisions about driving in chapter 45.)

Another safety concern relates to dyskinesia. Be careful to keep sharp objects off countertops where they might be knocked off.

Finally, and this seems like an obvious one, but many people do not set up their home to prevent falls. Things like removing scatter rugs, getting rid of clutter, widening doors, and installing grab bars can all help decrease the likelihood of your loved one having an accident. (You can read more about specific ways to Parkinson's-proof your home in chapter 25.)

Don't forget exercise

Exercise, exercise, exercise! You hear all the time—whether you have Parkinson's or not—that regular exercise is important. Well, it is. Studies have found that people who begin regular exercise early in the disease process experience a slower decline in their quality of life.[18] Doing 30 minutes of endurance exercise a day helps to maintain muscle control and tone and prevent rigidity.

In addition to helping minimize the symptoms of Parkinson's disease, exercise can be emotionally beneficial by helping alleviate depressed or anxious moods. Just the simple act of getting outside once a day to go for a walk or putter around the yard can loosen up muscles and diminish any depression your loved one might be experiencing.

To help your loved one stay motivated, consider exercising with them. The type of exercise you choose will depend on your loved one's symptoms, fitness level, and overall health. Generally, exercises that stretch the arms and legs through the full range of motion are encouraged.

Some ideas for exercise include walking, swimming, water aerobics (easier on the joints and requires less balance), yoga, and tai chi (both of which are relaxing and improve flexibility and balance).

Consider adjusting roles

As Parkinson's progresses, your loved one may no longer be able to take on the same responsibilities or perform the same household tasks they used to. For example, they may have difficulty managing finances, so you may have to take on this role. When it comes to physical tasks like yard work, you may want to consider hiring someone to do that.

Be careful when you go about making these changes, as your loved one may resist or be resentful. Talk things over with them and offer suggestions instead of telling them how things will or will not be.

Get help

As your loved one's Parkinson's progresses, they will have more needs to be met. As a caregiver, you will find that at some point, you won't be able meet all these needs. This is where building a caregiver team comes in handy. As I mentioned in chapter 3, getting help is one of (if not the most) important things you need to do while caring for your loved one.

The sooner you can start finding outside resources to help you, the better. Look for family or friends who can be your backup in case of an emergency or when you need a break.

Though the people on your caregiving team may play smaller roles for now, having them involved in your loved one's life early on will make it easier for them to fill in for you later when there's a greater need.

Watch for signs of caregiver stress

As Parkinson's progresses and your caregiving role evolves, you may find feelings of regret or resentment creeping in. It's okay to feel this way. Caregiving is a huge job, and especially difficult when you don't see an end in sight.

Throughout your caregiving journey, it's imperative that you care for yourself to make sure that you stay healthy and avoid getting burned out. You must know and respect your limits. Make it a priority to take regular breaks from caregiving, and when you are with your loved one, look for the things you love about your relationship.

Finally, don't forget that just because your loved one has Parkinson's doesn't mean that they can't take care of you a little. There are many acts of love, including a neck or foot massage, that are pretty easy to deliver through the mid-stages of Parkinson's disease.

24. Caregiving in the Late Stages of PD

"My advice to you is to do anything and everything that lifts the spirit and cheers the one who suffers from this disease. Nutrition is extremely important and a happy heart is a healing force. Never blame yourself and leave no stone unturned."

—Z, PARKINSON'S CAREGIVER

Quality. This is a word you'll often hear from health care providers as your loved one's Parkinson's advances into the late stages. The reason my mom designated me as power of attorney for her care was that she knew I would do my utmost to make sure she got the best quality of life for as long as she lived. I took this role very seriously, and with the help of a caregiver team, I believe I did a pretty good job.

If you've been caring for a loved one with Parkinson's through to the late stages of the disease, you've probably been serving in your role for a number of years. By now you've also probably experienced how exhausting this job can be, especially when it comes to providing physical care for your loved one.

As Parkinson's progresses into the late stages, you'll find that your loved one will need more help with daily activities such as walking, dressing, bathing, and getting in and out of a chair or bed. One key area to focus on will be taking advantage of your loved one's on periods and doing tasks during those times as much as possible. You may also have to dig deep into your patience jar, as many tasks will take your loved one longer to do than they used to.

Swallowing can become difficult in later stages so you may have to modify your loved one's diet to include only soft foods. See chapter 33 for more tips to help make swallowing easier.

Due to decreased mobility, your loved may also have challenges in getting food to their mouths, so you may want to try assistive devices such as double-handed cups to help them. See "Helpful

Gadgets for People With Parkinson's" in the appendix for more tools that may help make things easier for your loved one.

In addition to physical challenges, you will notice changes in your loved one's behavior, as well as in their thinking and memory. Dementia can also develop, and it is estimated that anywhere from 50 to 80 percent of people with Parkinson's have Parkinson's disease dementia (PDD).[19]

In the late stages of PD, your loved one may also experience hallucinations and delusions, which can be very scary for both of you (see chapter 30 for tips on dealing with those if they occur).

Even though many challenges accompany advanced Parkinson's, you can still do a lot to make your loved one's life easier, more comfortable, and more enjoyable. Keep in mind that word—*quality*. Focus on keeping your loved one safe and comfortable. Be patient and always remember to get help when you need it!

The chapters that follow in part 5 will provide the information you need to make things easier for you and your loved one as their disease progresses.

25. How to Parkinson's-Proof Your Home

"Never hide the fact that you suffer from PD. Wear this fact as a badge of honor." —ASH, PWP

If you're living in a home with someone with Parkinson's, you'll soon discover that various hazards around the house can make life difficult for them. Fortunately, there are some easy changes you can make to improve their safety.

To begin, start with smaller changes like decluttering your home and getting rid of potential obstacles—like scatter rugs and long cords on the floor. Creating clear pathways through your home can make mobility so much easier for someone with Parkinson's. The more open spaces you can create between furniture, the better.

Following are some more specific tips to help you make your home safer and "Parkinson's-proof."

All rooms
- Add more lights around the house. This can make it easier to navigate at all times of day. Consider touch- or voice-activated lights if these will be easier for your loved one to turn on and off.
- Create a contrasting pattern on the floor to help your loved one get from A to B more easily. In my mom's case, she had a friend cut out white squares (eight-by-eight-inch vinyl with an adhesive back) and stick them to the floor to create a pathway between the kitchen and the bathroom. When Mom needed to get from the kitchen to the bathroom and had trouble walking, she found that looking at the contrasting white squares on the floor helped her brain focus more on getting where she wanted to be. You can also

try adding stripes (about a foot apart) to the floor to help with walking.

Bathroom
- Get rid of bathmats that may slip and add a nonslip mat to the shower or bathtub.
- Install grab bars or safety rails beside or in front of the toilet. You may also want to look into getting an elevated toilet seat to make standing up easier.
- Install a horizontal grab bar along the sidewall above the tub and a vertical grab bar on the wall opposite the faucet to help with getting in and out. If using a shower stall, install grab bars or portable handles on the shower walls for balance when showering, as well as on the wall beside the toilet.
- If your bathroom has carpet, remove it. Depending on your budget you may also want to consider making the bathroom wheelchair accessible (e.g., widening the door, lowering the sink, building a shower that you can roll into with a chair).

Bedroom
- Put phones or emergency alarm systems in every room.
- Put night-lights in sockets to make it easier to navigate at night.
- Install a pole that stands beside the bed to help your loved one get in and out of it more easily. If you can't install a pole because your ceiling is high, you can install a wooden arm or grab bar on the wall. These devices can also help your loved one turn over in bed.
- If the bedroom is currently located a long way from the bathroom, you may want to consider moving it to a closer room to make getting to the bathroom that much easier (especially in the middle of the night).

- If it's in your budget, buy a bed with a control for raising and lowering its height.

Living room

- To avoid slipping and falling, get rid of scatter mats. Also, it is much easier to get around on hardwood or tiled floors than on carpet, so you may want to consider replacing carpets.
- Consider buying adjustable recliners or chairs with straight backs, firm seats, and armrests. This will make standing easier.
- Install railings along the walls and hallways to help with balance and to prevent falls.
- You may find that having an office chair on wheels in the house is handy as well. If you have hardwood or tiled floors, you can use this as a makeshift wheelchair for someone to push your loved one from point A to point B.

Kitchen

- Keep counters free of sharp knives. One time when Mom had a lot of dyskinesia, she accidentally knocked a knife off the counter and it braised her leg on the way down. As a caregiver, be aware of anything that could potentially be an accident waiting to happen in the kitchen!

Outside

- If it's in your budget, consider significant renovations such as ramps, stair lifts, and wider doorways.

26. Helping With Mobility

"My wife really finds relief in her weekly massage and has also completed a Pilate's course specifically aimed at improving balance and lengthening tendons, muscles, etc., to counteract the early indications." —CHRIS T., PARKINSON'S CAREGIVER

If you care for someone with Parkinson's, you're most likely already aware of their challenges with mobility. You can help your loved one with this in several ways. The first way is to understand how Parkinson's affects mobility.

When it comes to initiating first steps for walking, a person with Parkinson's may have problems lifting their feet and may have to take a few small and uneasy steps before walking at a steady pace. In addition, while walking, they may stop swinging their arms. You may also notice them shuffling their feet and walking with their weight on the balls of their feet.

The term "festinating gait" is used to describe when a person takes shorter than normal steps that become faster and faster. What sometimes happens is that the steps become so fast that the person falls forward or runs into something. Sometimes the same thing happens, only backward. There was a time when my mom had problems with this. For what seemed like no reason at all, she would start shuffling backward. We laughed at it to help her be less anxious and would say, "Hey, Mom, you need to switch gears. You're in reverse!"

You need to be careful as the caregiver if you see someone with Parkinson's shuffling because this can often lead to falls. About one-third of people with PD fall relatively frequently and lose their ability to regain their balance when they start to fall, so it is important to stay near them if they're having walking difficulties.

Something called freezing can also happen when a person with Parkinson's is walking. This often occurs in narrow spaces like doorways or when trying to turn. It basically makes it impossible for the person to move. It's like their feet are glued to the ground. You can read more about freezing and tips on helping the people you care for out of those sticky situations in the next chapter.

When it comes to increasing mobility with Parkinson's, the first step is to ask your loved one's doctor for an evaluation by a physical therapist. The therapist will draft a detailed evaluation with recommendations for treatment. Physical therapy can help people who are in various stages of Parkinson's, from the recently diagnosed to those who have had PD for many years. Though it can't stop the disease, it may help slow the loss of mobility that accompanies it. Physical therapists teach people with PD and their caregivers exercises to increase mobility and techniques to deal with specific trouble areas, such as freezing, getting in and out of bed, getting up from a seated position, and so forth.

My mom found physical therapy to be very helpful and had a physiotherapist visit her once a week in the early and mid-stages of her disease. She also tried to get outside every day to go for a walk. This was to help her keep her mobility for as long as possible (remember the saying "Move it or lose it!").

Sometimes when Mom's mobility wasn't great, she would push her wheelchair to help keep her balance and I, or a friend, would walk beside her, there to steady her in case she needed it.

As a caregiver, you will have to pay close attention to what works and what doesn't when it comes to keeping your loved one mobile. Sometimes walking while holding onto you will be better for them than, say, using a walker. One tip to remember is to let them hold onto you more than you hold onto them. This will give your loved one more confidence and allow them to decide when they want to let go.

Something else that Mom found helpful in terms of increasing her mobility was massage therapy. She loved massages and had them as often as she could.

If your loved one has trouble walking in the house, see if removing all their footwear (including slippery socks) helps. You don't want them wearing shoes that grip the floor and cause them to stumble. Mom found that making a barefoot connection with the floor made it easier for her to walk.

If your loved one has trouble walking through doorways (a common problem for people with PD), suggest that they try walking sideways, a trick that worked well for Mom.

As mentioned in the previous chapter, make clear pathways throughout your house to prevent tripping and falling at night. You may also want to install grab bars and railings along the walls, as well as night-lights.

Also mentioned in the previous chapter was the idea of creating contrasting patterns on the floor. The same principle can be applied outdoors. After we made a stone pathway (with pavers we got at the local hardware store) from her porch stairs to her garden, Mom was able to "follow the yellow brick road" (or white, in this case) to get to her garden without any problems. If your loved one is having mobility problems, a contrasting pattern on the floor or ground may be just the thing they need.

Another tip if your loved one is having trouble walking is to suggest that they try walking in a skating motion, sliding one foot at a time across the floor.

27. Managing Freezing Episodes

"I get started most easily if I imagine big, colored footprints leading forward from me, and then proceed to step on the footprints. It gets me going. Once I get going, I try to find my "natural" pace—one that is in tune with the frequency of a pendulum representing my body while walking. This pace I try to maintain so that I don't regress into a shuffle. For me, this "natural" pace is fairly brisk, like 3–4 mph. The imagining of footsteps is also useful when maneuvering to sit in a chair or negotiate through a crowd of people." —ROB F., PWP

One safety challenge that some people with Parkinson's face, especially those who are in the advanced stages or have been on the drug levodopa for a long time, is freezing. Freezing is the temporary, involuntary inability to move. For example, their feet may seem to stick to the floor, or they may be unable to get up from a chair.

It's important to note that although not everyone with PD will experience freezing, it can happen to anyone with the disease, not just those who take levodopa.

No one knows the exact cause of freezing, but it often happens when a person with Parkinson's is doing something and gets interrupted. For example, when they are walking and must make a turn or change direction. If this happens to your loved one, encourage them to make wider turns, and not in cramped spaces.

Another situation that can bring on freezing is being in crowded places, so avoiding these is ideal. Cluttered spaces can also be a challenge, so keeping your main living areas clean and tidy (keep chairs and other obstacles off to the side of the room) with enough room to move about is best.

Also, be aware that if your kitchen floor has a busy floral pattern on it like ours had, that can sometime cause freezing. You may want to consider redoing your flooring using either pattern-free tiles or a contrasting pattern (see chapter 25).

Finally, know that doorways can be a big freezing challenge. This proved to be the most common place where Mom would freeze, so we always made sure we were ready for it (see tips below). Freezing can be dangerous because it often leads to falls. As a caregiver, you mustn't try to force someone with PD to walk when they are in this state.

Though you may not always be able to prevent freezing, there are some things you can do to help your loved one through it.

- Count their steps out loud as they walk (try marching, or thinking "left, right, left, right . . .").
- One great thing Mom discovered was music. Play some fast-paced music (with a strong beat that you can march to) to keep your loved one going. Even better, carry a music player (iPod/smartphone) around with their favorite tunes so you can get them "plugged in" anytime they need a lift.
- Encourage your loved one to rock in place or shift their weight from foot to foot to get moving again.
- Place your foot in front of your loved one or ask them to visualize something they need to step over.
- Try using a LaserCane. This cane projects a bright red line across your path, which acts as a visual cue to help break freezing episodes and increase stride length.
- Suggest that your loved one cover their eyes. This can trick their brain and allow them to walk straight ahead with no problems.
- If your loved one is in a hurry they can slowly sink to their knees and crawl, but obviously this is only practical at home.
- Suggest walking very carefully backward or sideways. (This worked very well for Mom, especially when she needed to walk through a doorway.)
- They may choose to simply wait—after all, the freezing will pass.

28. Preventing Falls

"The advice I had from our occupational therapist was to have a walk-in shower installed and grab rails fitted in the bathtub for my husbands' safety." —JOY, PARKINSON'S CAREGIVER

Unfortunately, because of the nature of Parkinson's and how it affects balance and stability, people with this disease are prone to falling. Falls become more common as the disease progresses. In fact, up to two-thirds of people with Parkinson's experience falls each year (compared to a third of the general elderly population).

Falls in PD occur mostly when turning or changing directions and are often related to a freezing episode. People with Parkinson's might also experience falls as a result of orthostatic hypotension (postural low blood pressure) and problems with vision.

There is no single solution to preventing falls in PD, and because they become more and more common as people age, the main focus should be on preventing frequent falls and minimizing injury.

As a caregiver, one big thing you can do to help keep your loved one from falling is to make your home safer. Tips on how to do this were mentioned in chapter 25 on home safety for people with Parkinson's.

Here are some more specific tips to help with fall prevention.

- Ensure that your loved one takes their medication as prescribed to reduce the severity of motor symptoms.
- Help your loved one stay focused while walking by avoiding distractions. Even talking can contribute to falls, as multitasking may be hard for the Parkinson's brain.
- To increase muscle strength, stability, and balance, have your loved one try an exercise and physical therapy program individually tailored to their needs.
- Make sure your loved one is wearing appropriate footwear to help them move around more easily and keep them more

stable (ladies, put away your heels!). Mom found that walking around barefoot was best for her while in the house.

- Encourage your loved one to always keep one hand free to grab onto surrounding objects and/or break the force of a fall if need be.
- Consider withdrawal of psychotropic medications.
- Always seek medical attention, even after a minor fall, to identify the full extent of injuries and have them treated immediately to limit complications.

If your loved one with PD is in a care facility, you may want to consider the following for additional help in preventing falls.

- Use of vitamin D and calcium supplements
- Use of hip protectors

Studies have shown that there is no evidence to support the effectiveness of interventions to reduce falls among people with cognitive impairments. In addition, using physical or pharmaceutical restraints has not been found to prevent falls. In fact, there is some evidence to support an increased risk of injury from a fall with the use of restraints.[20]

29. Getting the Most Out of Medications

"I think that everyone should know about the possible side effects of higher doses of Mirapex. My husband had been online gambling for ten months to a year before I found out. We lost over $160,000 to gambling. The connection was the amount of Mirapex he was taking. When the doctor lowered the dosage, the desire went away for my husband. He had no prior interest in gambling until the doses increased. I hope this will help others before it is too late." —LISA, PARKINSON'S CAREGIVER

As a caregiver for someone with Parkinson's, you'll soon discover how necessary medications are in their daily lives. Making sure that they get their medications on time is one of the most important things you can do for them throughout their Parkinson's journey. Doing so will give them the best chance of managing their symptoms throughout the day. Parkinson's medications aren't cheap, either, making it very important that your loved one get the most out of each dose.

Following are some tips to increase the effectiveness of Parkinson's medications.

- Take the medication as prescribed by their doctor. Make sure you understand the expected benefit and potential early side effects of a drug before you and your loved one leave the doctor's office. Remember that the doctor probably has more clinical experience in treating people with PD than anyone else who is likely to give you advice.
- Do not increase or suddenly stop any drugs without checking with their doctor first.
- Levodopa generally works best on an empty stomach, so aim to take meds around a half hour before meals, or at

least an hour after. However, if medication is causing your loved one to feel nauseous, they may have to take it with food until their body adjusts.

- Make sure meds are taken with four to five ounces of water so that the drugs are absorbed quickly.

A tip my mom shared was to avoid eating large amounts of protein at any one time. She found that eating too much protein really reduced the effectiveness of her meds (specifically levodopa).

Another tip Mom had for helping medications work better is to avoid sitting in one place for long periods of time. If you have to sit anywhere for more than an hour, encourage your loved one to get up every hour and do some stretching or moving around to keep their muscles from stiffening up too much. Mom said that regardless of when she last took her medications, sitting in one spot for a long time made it hard to get moving again.

Though you may not always be able to achieve it, you should be aiming for as little off time (the time when your loved one basically has to stay put because your medications have worn off) as possible.

Most people with Parkinson's find that after they take their meds, there is a wait time before they kick in. Wait times are commonly 20 to 30 minutes, but because everyone is different this can vary, and it can depend on everything from how long a person has had the disease to what they last ate. In Mom's case, she had to wait for up to 45 minutes (often less than this) after she took her medications for them to start working and for her to have on time (or in her words, for her to "have wheels").

My mom's way of telling whether she was getting the most out of her meds was to see how much time each day she spent in off mode. If she had to wait more than an hour for her meds to kick in or had more than four hours in one day in off time, she knew she needed to talk to her doctor about possibly changing the dosage and/or timing of her medications. (*Note:* It can be helpful for your loved one's doctor to know exactly when they are experiencing on and off times, as well as dyskinesia if they experience that, so that the doctor may better prescribe their daily meds regimen. I've included a "PD ON/OFF Diary" in the free resources section of AllAboutParkinsons.com that will help you keep track of when your loved one is at their best each day.)

One thing that helped maximize the effectiveness of my mom's meds was that she was able to take them on an empty stomach. This wasn't possible for her in the beginning because she got nauseous all the time when she took her meds (a common side effect of the drugs). But after her body got used to her medications, she was able to switch the timing. A tip she shared to reduce nausea is to take meds with crackers, juice, or ginger ale.

Mom said the good thing about having less food in your stomach is that the meds work better, but sometimes it seems that they are working too well because you get more of the medication side effect dyskinesia. You might have to experiment a bit with the timing of meals and meds to find out what works best for your loved one.

In case you or your loved one is admitted to a hospital, know that most hospitals organize medication administration around standardized times and allow medications to be given 30 minutes before or after these times. It's up to you to let them know that PD medications should be given on your schedule, not theirs.

30. How to Deal With Hallucinations and Delusions

"The greatest challenge I have had as caregiver is the fact that I was pretty much prepared for his becoming more and more dependent on me as far as his physical condition worsened, but I was not prepared and had not been told before that the Parkinson's and the medicine could cause hallucinations. That has been his problem also, because he is constantly seeing things and people that are real to him but that I do not see."

—MARGE, PARKINSON'S CAREGIVER

Here is something I did not know about Parkinson's when my mom was first diagnosed: people with this disease can experience hallucinations and delusions. Fortunately, not everyone with PD experiences these often-frightening symptoms. Those who do are usually older and have had the disease for a long time. Hallucinations and delusions may be caused in part by the disease and in part by the Parkinson's medications.

A hallucination is when you think that something is there that it isn't. A delusion is when you are convinced that something is true despite clear evidence proving that it is not.

Types of hallucinations
- Visual hallucinations (seeing things that aren't there)
- Auditory hallucinations (hearing things that aren't there)
- Tactile hallucinations (sensing things that aren't there)

Types of delusions
- Paranoia (e.g., thinking someone is following you when they aren't)
- Jealousy (thinking people you love are betraying you)
- Extravagance (believing you have special powers)

Mom experienced visual hallucinations in the late stages of her disease. Sometimes her hallucinations were scary (e.g., she thought there was a big black hole in front of her that her grandkids kept falling into), while other times not (e.g., her deceased husband was sitting in her room with her).

Through trial and error, we figured out that these hallucinations and delusions were mostly a side effect of a drug (amantadine) that she took for her dyskinesia. At first we tried reassuring her that what she was seeing wasn't real. This helped calm her down initially. However, as the hallucinations got worse and she became more frightened by them, we opted for medication changes.

It was a delicate balance trying to keep her dyskinesia to a minimum while warding off hallucinations. By reducing (not eliminating) the meds she took for dyskinesia, the hallucinations mostly stopped until she passed.

If your loved one experiences hallucinations or delusions, you should encourage them to talk with you about them. This will help you to better support them and understand what they are going through.

If the hallucinations/delusions are not frightening and your loved one is aware that they are not real, they may choose to live with this side effect. If, on the other hand, your loved one is frightened, you will want to talk with their doctor to find possible solutions. The doctor will check for other causes of these symptoms. Things like an imbalance of chemicals in the blood; improper kidney, liver, or lung function; and certain infections can cause these mental disturbances.

Other medications that your loved one may be taking, including over-the-counter meds, could also be responsible. Make sure that you tell the doctor about all medications, including herbal therapies, your loved one is taking.

If no other causes for the hallucinations or delusions are found, the doctor may choose to make adjustments to the Parkinson's medications. Some people may not be able to tolerate changes in their PD meds without the worsening of their symptoms. In these cases, it may be necessary to treat the mental disturbances with antipsychotic medications. Unfortunately, some of these can worsen PD symptoms. There are alternatives, though, and the doctor will be able to help you find them if needed.

31. How to Handle Weight Loss

"When my (6'1") dad got down to 139 lbs., I went ballistic. The doctor finally took me seriously and put Dad on an appetite enhancing drink called Megace. He got one drink in the morning and one at night. I had to discontinue the one at night because he was literally up all night eating. He has gained 16 lbs. in two months and for whatever reason is enjoying his food. He is gaining strength and his bowels are so much better because he is getting volume. It is the single best thing I have done."

—MELODY, PARKINSON'S CAREGIVER

Many people with Parkinson's lose weight after diagnosis. It's a fairly common problem, especially for women. My mom had issues with this in the later stages of her disease and it was a bit of a challenge coming up with the perfect diet to keep her from losing weight.

Researchers aren't entirely sure why this happens. Some think it may be that people with PD eat less due to loss of appetite caused by depression, or loss of sense of smell. Others think it could be all the shaking and dyskinesia associated with the disease or the swallowing problems that cause people with Parkinson's to lose weight.

Whatever the reason behind weight loss in PD, it can have some serious side effects in your loved one, including a weakened immune system, muscle loss, and loss of important nutrients. If you find your loved one can't stop the weight from coming off, there are several things you can do to help them. Consult with their doctor if you think any of the following tips will help.

Maintaining a healthy weight
- Weigh your loved one once or twice a week, unless their doctor recommends weighing more often. If your loved one is taking diuretics or steroids, you should weigh daily.
- If they have an unexplained weight gain or loss (two pounds in one day or five pounds in one week), talk to their

106

doctor. He or she may want to change food or fluid intake to help manage the condition.

Gaining weight

- Ask your loved one's doctor about nutritional supplements. Sometimes supplements in the form of snacks, drinks, or vitamins may be prescribed for consumption between meals to help increase caloric intake and get the right amount of nutrients every day. Just make sure you look for high-calorie—*not* high-protein—drink supplements. Also, have them avoid taking medications with these supplements.
- Avoid low-fat or low-calorie products (unless their doctor has recommended otherwise).

Note: Make sure you check with the doctor before making any dietary changes or before adding supplements to your loved one's diet. Some can be harmful or interfere with Parkinson's medications.

Improving a poor appetite

- Sometimes poor appetite is due to depression, which can be treated. Talk to the doctor if this applies to your loved one. Their desire to eat will probably improve after depression is treated.
- Avoid nonnutritious drinks like soda.
- Have them eat small, frequent meals and snacks.
- If your loved one is able, encourage them to walk or get involved in another light activity to stimulate their appetite.
- Ask the doctor about potential appetite-enhancing drinks that may be prescribed.

Eating more at meals

- Have drinks after a meal instead of before or during to prevent your loved one from feeling full before they start eating or to fill up too quickly.

- Choose foods that are a different color than the plate. People with Parkinson's can develop vision changes, with the amount of contrast sensitivity in the eye making it hard to discern objects that are similar in color. Try using dark-colored dishes when serving light-colored foods and light-colored dishes when serving dark-colored foods.
- Plan meals to include their favorite foods.
- Try eating the high-calorie foods in a meal first.
- Increase the variety of food (use your imagination or a good cookbook).

Snacking

- Choose high-calorie snacks, ideally those with some nutritional value. Try peanut butter and toast, nachos with guacamole and a protein, or an omelet.
- Make food preparation easy. Choose foods that are easy to make and eat.
- Make eating a pleasant experience, not a chore. To liven things up at mealtimes, try putting on background music and using colorful place settings.
- As much as possible, eat with your loved one so that they aren't eating alone. If you're not around for a while, encourage them to invite somebody over for dinner or to go out.

If your loved one is having weight loss problems and is living in a nursing home, you may have to be extra diligent in helping them get the nutrition they need. Ask to meet with the on-site dietician (most homes have one; if not then ask to speak to your loved one's doctor) to discuss options to keep your loved one eating. Don't give up until you get the help you're looking for!

32. Help for Drooling and Dry Mouth

"I had a major problem with an extremely dry mouth while sleeping at night (possibly due to the Mirapex I take before bedtime). My doctor recommended rinsing my mouth with Biotene mouthwash (a 'Mouthwash for Dry Mouth Care') before going to bed, and it really made a difference. It is available at any drugstore and has a very pleasant taste."

—ANONYMOUS, PWP

If your loved one has problems with drooling, they may have experienced the embarrassment that it can cause. As their caregiver, you may have felt some of this embarrassment too.

People with Parkinson's may have more saliva than people without the disease because they swallow less often and because they may produce more saliva in general. As a result of this excess amount of saliva, drooling (also called sialorrhea) is often the result. Drooling can not only be annoying and sometimes embarrassing, it can also be dangerous as swallowing saliva into your lungs can cause pneumonia.

There are several things you can do to help prevent drooling (see tips below), but if they either don't work or stop working, your loved one will have to talk to their doctor. He or she may prescribe anticholinergic drugs or sometimes recommend Botox (botulinum toxin) injections. When Botox is injected into the salivary glands, the results can last several months.

Fortunately there are some things that can be done to prevent drooling. Encourage your loved one to try some of the tips below.

- Suck on hard candy, lozenges, or chew gum (ideally sugarless) to control excess saliva (if they are not at risk of choking).

- Use a straw to help strengthen their lip, mouth, and throat muscles.
- Try to keep their head up and posture straight because stooping encourages drooling.
- Swallow first before talking.
- When they're not eating or talking, keep their mouth closed and lips tight together (people with PD tend to let their jaw drop open, which encourages drooling).
- Breathe through their nose (this will help keep their mouth closed, which will then help keep the saliva in their mouth).
- Swallow to help prevent saliva buildup.
- Try rubbing a strong-smelling lip balm over their mouth to remind them to swallow.
- Put one or two drops of atropine eye drops (0.5%) under their tongue to reduce the amount of saliva. (This works for some people, but they should check with their doctor first.)

Dry mouth

Though less common than drooling, dry mouth can be a problem for people with Parkinson's and may be related to PD medications. Dry mouth can feel uncomfortable and also lead to teeth and mouth decay. (Saliva acts as an antibacterial, and less of it means less protection against decay.)

Tips to help your loved one with dry mouth
- Consult with their doctor as you may need to make changes in their medications.
- If they are not at risk of choking, suggest sucking on hard candies or chewing gum to help keep their mouth lubricated. Eating sour candy can also increase saliva production and help to moisten their mouth.
- Reduce consumption of dry foods like peanut butter, crackers, and chips, because they stick to the throat and dry out the mouth.

- Soften foods by adding liquid (e.g., gravy, broth, sauce, or melted butter) or by dunking them in liquids (e.g., dipping cookies or crackers in milk, coffee, or tea).
- Drink between bites to moisten their mouth and help them swallow.
- Breathe through their nose instead of their mouth.
- If they smoke, encourage them to cut down or even quit because this can be a major factor in drying out their mouth and causing gum problems.
- Try taking a cotton swab dipped in olive oil and rubbing it on the inside of their mouth every hour or so.
- Don't use a commercial mouthwash that contains alcohol. Their doctor or dentist will be able to provide a recommendation for an alternative that will not cause dry mouth.
- Ask their doctor or dentist about prescription toothpaste (higher fluoride content).
- Limit their caffeine intake. Caffeine is a diuretic, meaning it can make them thirstier and cause them to urinate more frequently, resulting in dehydration.
- Consider an artificial saliva product, but ask their doctor about this first.
- Keep hydrated. For most people, eight glasses a day is a good rule of thumb. However, if your loved one has a heart problem, consult with their doctor about their fluid intake; the doctor may recommend limiting their fluids depending on their condition.

33. Mealtime and Swallowing Tips

"We ordered some foam-handled cutlery (for dad), which makes eating so much easier." —KRISTEN K., PARKINSON'S CAREGIVER

Having difficulties swallowing (a condition called dysphagia) can happen at any stage of Parkinson's, though it's more common in the later stages. Problems with chewing and swallowing solid foods is a common symptom resulting from, among other factors, the loss of muscle control in the jaw and throat. Another contributing factor is that people with PD often bend their neck when they sit, which forces them to look down. This makes it hard for their jaw to work properly to chew and swallow.

Challenges with swallowing may cause your loved one to cough or choke while they're eating, or they may find themselves drooling. Over time, issues with swallowing can also lead to weight loss. If you are noticing these symptoms in your loved one, contact their doctor. He or she may be able to recommend a speech pathologist who can help your loved one learn new techniques for chewing and swallowing.

My mom periodically used to cough when she ate, and usually it reminded her to be more focused on what she was doing (and use some of the tips below). Thankfully she only once had a choking episode where food got stuck in her throat and she couldn't swallow for a few seconds (I quickly gave her the Heimlich maneuver to dislodge the food). In the later stages of PD, Mom ate only softer (and sometimes pureed) foods that she didn't have to chew much.

Suggestions to help your loved one chew and swallow more easily
- Sit upright at a 90-degree angle (one way they can do this is to straddle their chair).
- Tilt their head slightly forward.

- Sit with their elbows on the table, which forces their spine, neck, and chin up.
- Keep the distractions to a minimum in the area where they eat.
- Eat slowly and avoid talking when there is food in their mouth.
- Prepare small bites of food and chew carefully and thoroughly (no more than one-half teaspoon of food per bite).
- Remain upright up for 15 to 20 minutes after a meal.
- If they are struggling to swallow or food or liquids are catching in their throat, try swallowing multiple times per bite or sip. When something feels stuck, clear their throat or cough gently and then try swallowing one more time before taking a breath. Repeat this as necessary.
- Increase saliva production and swallowing frequency by sucking on popsicles, ice chips, lemon ice, or lemon-flavored water.
- Try eating softer foods that require less chewing. You can also puree their meals in a blender to achieve this effect.
- Swap thin liquids for thick ones (e.g., cream soup for broth) as thin liquids may make them cough. They can also use a liquid thickener (their speech pathologist can recommend one).
- Ask their doctor about crushing their pills and mixing them with applesauce or pudding. *Do not do this without consulting their doctor or pharmacist first!* While this may help with swallowing, crushing pills can alter how the PD medication works.
- Your loved one may be able to take their levodopa/carbidopa in the form of Parcopa, which dissolves in their mouth.

34. Social and Activity Concerns

"My husband had impeccable table manners and even abhorred others that gulped down their food and otherwise expressed poor table etiquette. Now he does things at the table that are downright embarrassing. If I try to correct him, much like a child, he gets offended and angry. But I can't just let him destroy the table and its contents."

—ANONYMOUS, PARKINSON'S CAREGIVER

People with Parkinson's report the number one challenge to living well with the disease is stigma. Because of this, those with PD are particularly vulnerable to withdrawing from their favorite activities and adopting a less physically active lifestyle. Also, the loss of dopamine in their brains impacts their self-efficacy (their belief that they can succeed at an activity), which can lead to anxiety, depression, and fatigue.

As the disease progresses, it can be hard for a person with PD to be in public. It took some time before my mom was able to stop thinking that people were looking at her like she was a freak, with all the moving and shaking she did. Also, my mom would often have trouble walking through doorways and experienced a sudden shutdown of her body. This often attracted attention from others and was emotionally disturbing for her.

As their caregiver, try to ignore any unwanted attention your loved one may be receiving. Though it may be hard for both of you at first, over time you will develop ways to deal with different social situations.

Sometimes when Mom and I were out shopping, I would tell the salesperson about her having Parkinson's. Each time I did, we received nothing but help and empathy. You may or may not choose to do this, but I have found that most people are afraid of what they don't know, so helping them to understand a bit about Parkinson's helps.

Eating out can also be challenging for a person with PD because they can have trouble holding onto cutlery or cups. Several times my mom ended up embarrassed and upset because she couldn't stop dropping things and spilling food at the dinner table. Even among friends, she often found eating very emotionally difficult.

A couple of things we did to help Mom feel less embarrassed while eating out was to carry a pretty scarf and a clip that we could attach to her shirt (a fancy bib) and bring our own utensils that were easier for her to grasp.

Social isolation can be a problem for those with PD, and as a caregiver you need to pay attention to your loved one for signs of withdrawal. Social connection is an essential part of your loved one's treatment, and helping them feel needed can make a huge difference in their life with PD.

Dr. Laurie Mischley, a naturopathic physician who runs a clinical practice for people with Parkinson's out of Seattle, has been conducting a study to determine the key factors in the progression of PD. Out of all the data her team has looked at so far, answering yes to the statement "I am lonely" is the single biggest predictor of Parkinson's progression.[21]

If your loved one is able, there are several ways you can help them feel needed. You can encourage them to participate or volunteer their time for a Parkinson's function (e.g., Parkinson's SuperWalk, Pancakes for Parkinson's), volunteer for their church or favorite charity, or sign up for a class (art, music, language, etc.) that meets every week. My mom volunteered once a week for her local Alzheimer's association (her dad had the disease) in the early stages of her PD and found that to be very fulfilling.

Another thing you can do to promote socialization and exercise at the same time is to encourage your loved one to join a specialized exercise class such as Rock Steady Boxing, Pedaling for Parkinson's, yoga, or tai chi class. If you really want to be supportive, consider joining in with them! Group classes offer new social connections, can help your loved one overcome barriers, and increase their quality of life all at the same time.

PART 6

Especially for Spouses

35. Special Needs of Spousal Caregivers

"The most important thing I can tell people is never forget that the person you are now taking care of is still that man/woman you fell in love with. Never let them doubt for a minute that you still think of them in that manner. Cherish them in all aspects. Make sure they know early on that during the times you become frustrated as a caregiver (and you will) you aren't frustrated with them, but with the darned disease."

—SHARRON H., PARKINSON'S CAREGIVER

"In sickness and in health . . ." As a spousal caregiver, this vow may mean a lot more than you ever thought it would. If so, you may feel better knowing that there are millions of others out there just like you. According to the National Family Caregivers Association, 1 in 10 caregivers in America are caring for a spouse.[22]

Caring for a spouse with Parkinson's can be emotionally draining and stressful. It can be hard shifting from spouse to caregiver, and you may not know how to deal with the challenges that come with the new role. You may also have to deal with feelings of loneliness in your relationship, isolation from friends, and resentment or anger toward your spouse. If your loved one has dementia in addition to Parkinson's, you will also have to deal with a greater sense of loss.

With all this on your plate, you must make sure your needs are being met. In fact, caring for yourself can be one of the most important things you to do help your loved one. It can help you maintain your marriage while you shift into the caregiver role, and also help prevent stress and burnout, which will enable you to provide better care.

Failing to take care of your needs can lead to a decline in your own health and even increase your risk of death. Studies have found that older spousal caregivers have a significantly higher risk (over 60 percent) of dying than do their non-caregiving peers if they experience ongoing mental and emotional strain.[23]

There are many ways to take care of yourself that are discussed throughout this book. Two key things to remember are to allow others to help you (caregiving is not a solo job) and to take regular breaks.

36. What to Do When Your Life Becomes All About Parkinson's

"My husband has had Parkinson's disease for 11 years. He is 58 years old and getting into advanced stages now. Our whole life is Parkinson's: about how he doesn't sleep and his foot cramps; all his medicine he has to take. That's most of our conversations, and it's getting very depressing for me. I have tried to tell him to talk about something different and now I have given up on this matter. It wears me down. Please help!"

—ANONYMOUS, PARKINSON'S CAREGIVER

Unfortunately, the above sentiment expressed by a Parkinson's caregiver is quite common. It's especially common among spousal caregivers, as they spend most, if not all, of their time with their loved one.

If you've been caring for your loved one for some time, Parkinson's can end up consuming your life. If Parkinson's is taking over your life, there are steps you can take to regain balance.

Know yourself

Remember this mantra: "Caregiving is something you do—it's not who you are." Though caregiver may be one of your roles, it's important to realize and remind yourself that you have other roles as well. In my case, I am also a wife, a daughter, a sister, an aunt, a friend, a swimmer, and a writer, among other things.

If you dig deeper, you'll find that I'm sensitive and empathetic to those in need (in particular, the elderly), and I tend to wear my heart on my sleeve. I'm also analytical, super competitive, and very passionate about a lot of things.

Take some time to think about who you are and the roles you play in your life. Knowing yourself will enable you to figure out what your limits are, as well as decide what you feel comfortable with and how much you are willing to give in your caregiving role.

Set boundaries

I talked about setting boundaries already (see chapter 4), but it's worth repeating how necessary they are. As a spouse caring for someone with Parkinson's, there may be assumptions that you do everything. Friends, family, even doctors and nurses may say, "Don't worry, the wife/husband will do it." Sometimes people assume that because you're the spouse, you should be prepared and willing to do everything that needs to be done.

It's okay to express that you're overwhelmed in your caregiving role. We all have limits, and as a spousal caregiver, you don't—and shouldn't—have to do it all. Setting boundaries with which you are comfortable is an essential step in ensuring that you are able to be the best caregiver you can be. Talk to your spouse about how you're feeling, and in a loving and caring way, discuss what you are and aren't willing and able to do.

Set goals

It's easy to put your life on hold while you're immersed in a caregiving role. The problem is that you probably won't know how long your life will be on hold. In the meantime, you could lose out on many opportunities.

Having goals can help make life more exciting and give you something to strive for. To help you achieve your goals, make sure you are consistently working on them. Even if it's for only 15 minutes a day, you'll find that your goals gain momentum if you stick with them consistently over time.

Ask your spouse to give, not just receive

If you're caring for your spouse, you may find that the give and take in your relationship has become very imbalanced as time goes on. One of the things to remember is that your loved one is capable of giving back, even if it's just in small ways. If they can't help around the house or do tasks that they used to, you can remind them that they can still listen to you and express their gratitude, both of which can go a long way in your relationship.

Reconnect with your spouse

It's easy for a marriage to get lost in Parkinson's. Your social time together may be hampered, especially if you have a partner with PD who can no longer do the things you used to do together (for instance, going out dancing). Finding new activities that you both can do is the key here. Allow yourself to simply be with your partner instead of focusing on what needs to be done all the time.

If you find this hard to do, consider giving up caregiving tasks that may be more demanding or that cause stress in your relationship. Hiring someone to come in to take the load off you can enable you to focus on spending more quality time with your spouse.

Always remember: Don't let Parkinson's get between you and your spouse!

37. When Parkinson's Is Keeping You Up All Night

"The bedside rail has been a wonderful tool. My mother hasn't slipped off the side of the bed since we purchased the rail."

—ANONYMOUS, PARKINSON'S CAREGIVER

Parkinson's disease creates many challenges with respect to getting a good night's sleep. In fact, it has been estimated that up to 96 percent of those with PD experience sleep difficulties of some kind.[24] If you're caring for a spouse with Parkinson's, their sleep problems will most likely affect the quality of your sleep as well.

Problems with sleep include insomnia, disrupted sleep, acting out dreams (also called REM behavior disorder, very common in PD), nightmares, vivid dreaming, sleepwalking (not very common), sleep talking, sleep apnea (when breathing stops for a few seconds), excessive daytime sleepiness (EDS), nocturia (waking up with the urge to urinate), and restless legs syndrome (RLS).

There are many possible reasons for sleep problems in people with Parkinson's. One of the more common ones is medication. People with PD can often have problems falling asleep or staying asleep when their meds (e.g., levodopa or dopamine agonists) start to wear off before the next dose is due. This causes symptoms such as tremor, rigidity, pain, and turning over in bed.

The antiparkinsonian medications amantadine and selegiline can also make it hard for people to fall asleep or stay asleep, due to their stimulant effect. My mom had this problem. With advanced Parkinson's, she would sometimes experience excessive dyskinesia, which she took amantadine to control. Though the amantadine did work to calm her body, unfortunately it also tended to keep her awake, sometimes the entire night.

Other medications can be responsible for sleep disruptions. Diuretics (to promote urine production and flow) can be at fault.

If they are not taken early enough in the day your loved one may have to get up a lot during the night to go to the bathroom.

The drug ephedrine (a stimulant used to treat postural hypotension) can also disrupt sleep. And keep in mind that over-the-counter pills like decongestants and antihistamines may cause sleep problems as well.

Food is another common—and often overlooked—culprit. Stimulants make falling asleep and staying asleep more difficult. Avoid the caffeine rush from consuming tea, coffee, and chocolate. Alcohol is another one to steer clear of; while initially a depressant that makes you sleepy, it can ultimately act as a stimulant and cause you to wake up during the second half of the sleep period.

Anxiety, depression, and other psychological problems (including dementia) are also causes of insomnia and sleep disturbances.

As a spouse, you can help your partner by learning more about their individual problems with sleep and consulting with their doctor to find ways to improve their quality and quantity of sleep.

Before you go in for your appointment, look for patterns in your loved one's sleep disturbance. Did you notice that it became worse after they started a new medication? Taking medications at different times may help difficulties with sleep, but it may take some time to figure out when the best times are. Their doctor can help determine this, and whether they need to change the dosage before bedtime. Does your loved one always have painful cramping at a certain time of night? Do they notice that certain foods or drinks make it worse? The more specific the information you can provide their doctor, the better.

Here are some tips that may help your loved one enjoy more comfortable, restful sleep.

For problems moving or turning in bed
- Try side rails, a trapeze, ropes, or a handle to grip.
- Use satin sheets or pajamas. (Mom said satin sheets are the best!)

- Change to a firmer, lower, or higher mattress.
- Consult a physical or occupational therapist.

For foot and leg sensitivity in bed

- Take the pressure off feet and legs. A bed hoop or a blanket cradle can be useful, or an electric blanket or light down comforter might provide enough relief.

For restless legs, painful cramping, or abnormal movements

- Talk to your loved one's doctor because he or she may change medication times or dosages or order other medications for pain, spasm, cramps, or anxiety.
- Try relaxation techniques or slow, relaxing stretching exercises.
- Walk around to help relieve RLS.

For frequent urination at night

- Talk to your loved one's doctor or urologist to correct issues such as prostate problems, urinary retention, or infections.
- Put a urinal or commode near the bedside.

For fear of falling at night

- Make your home safer by getting rid of scatter rugs and using night-lights.
- Try using a walker at night if able.
- To prevent dizziness, don't get up too quickly.

For shortness of breath or heartburn

- Using extra pillows or support blocks to raise the head of the bed may help reduce these symptoms, but both symptoms should be discussed with your doctor.

For excessive daytime sleepiness (EDS)

- Talk to your doctor if your loved one is taking antidepressants, as he or she may change the times or dosages of your medications.
- Be very careful when driving, operating machinery, or doing any other activity that requires alertness.
- Insufficient or poor-quality sleep at night can cause EDS, so addressing the quality and amount of nighttime sleep can help.

Another tip you may want to consider is sleeping in side-by-side twin beds, or even in separate rooms, to ensure better rest for both of you. If you decide to sleep in separate rooms, your loved one could use a call button, alert system, or monitor to let you know if they need help.

38. How Can I Regain Respect for My Spouse With PD?

"How can I get the respect back that I had for my husband before he became ill with Parkinson's? With his constant dribbling and incontinence issues I do struggle even though I know that it is not his fault. Luckily, I am able to still leave him on his own sometimes during the day to regain my sanity but as soon as I return, the feeling returns. I hate myself for feeling this way."

—ANONYMOUS, PARKINSON'S CAREGIVER

When your role of wife or husband has shifted to caregiver, there are many challenges you will face, including some that may be difficult for you to admit. Losing respect for the person you married is one challenge that can arise, especially in the late stages of the disease.

If you're struggling with this, don't beat yourself up about it. Recognizing when your feelings toward your spouse have changed can spur you on to take steps toward regaining respect for them.

Though it may not always be easy, there are some things you can do to let your spouse know you still respect them.

- Know it's not their fault. Remember that it is Parkinson's—*not* them—that is making your spouse act or feel a certain way.
- Find something you respect about your spouse. Even if it is something as small as your spouse smelling nice, let them know you respect that about them and affirm them for it.
- Show them love and affection. Remember that your spouse is not Parkinson's. Though they may have symptoms that neither of you enjoy, they are still the person you married and need you to be close to them when they are suffering.
- Know and accept your spouse's limitations. Living with Parkinson's can be frustrating and depressing at times.

Don't make things worse by unintentionally setting up
your spouse for failure by expecting them to do things
they can't do.

- Educate yourself about Parkinson's. Parkinson's affects every
  aspect of life, so the more you know, the more supportive
  and compassionate you can be toward your spouse.
- Avoid dwelling on what could have been. Nothing in life
  is for certain, so accept your situation and make the best
  of it. Look for and talk about the things for which you are
  thankful. Find things you can both look forward to and set
  reachable goals together.
- Talk to your spouse and encourage them to talk to you
  about the way they are feeling. What does your spouse need
  more or less of? Let them know what your needs are as well.
- Avoid scolding and criticizing your spouse. Good things
  never come from doing either of these.
- Don't patronize or talk down to them. This sometimes
  happens when a loved one develops dementia and starts
  behaving like someone much younger than they are. Resist
  doing this; instead, be kind and reassuring.
- Respect your spouse's privacy and be sensitive if they need
  help with personal activities like washing or going to
  the toilet.
- Take a break together. Find a mutual interest outside of
  Parkinson's— something you can both enjoy—and do it! It
  could be something as simple as going for a walk, reading
  together, or watching a funny movie at home. Having a
  life together outside of Parkinson's will make your marriage
  both stronger and happier.
- Know that it's okay to get emotional. It's not easy to live
  with and care for a spouse with Parkinson's, and it may cost
  you a lot of emotional energy. Give yourself permission to
  feel the things you are feeling as you face caregiving challenges. Find a friend or professional to whom you can talk
  when you're feeling overwhelmed, frustrated, angry, or sad.

This will help you stay emotionally healthy and in the best shape to support your spouse.

Remember, if you want to be the best caregiver for your spouse, understanding what it's like to live with PD is imperative. Always try to appreciate how they feel, and do your best to support and reassure them. Being compassionate toward them will be a win-win for both of you!

39. Parkinson's and Your Sex Life

"If your doctor doesn't suggest it, help yourself out by looking into the many alternative treatments that are available today. And, by all means, join the Well Spouse Association. Their newsletter, *Mainstay*, can be a lifesaver for the spousal caregiver."

—AMIE, PARKINSON'S CAREGIVER

Many spouses caring for someone with Parkinson's have difficulties talking about the topic of sex and for good reason: it's a sensitive and sometimes uncomfortable and embarrassing subject. As you've been caring for your loved one with PD, you may or may not have encountered the problems the disease can cause with respect to your sex life, such as a decreased sex drive, hypersexuality, or difficulties with arousal.

Decreased dopamine levels may cause a decrease in sex drive in Parkinson's brains, but it is more likely a result of stress, anxiety, and depression in the aftermath of diagnosis. And many people with depression are prescribed antidepressants, which themselves often decrease libido.

On the opposite end of the spectrum are those who experience hypersexuality, an impulsive and compulsive behavior in which people find themselves preoccupied with sexual feelings and thoughts. Hypersexuality can be a side effect of dopamine agonists (and sometimes levodopa), so if it becomes an issue, a change of meds may be needed. Ask your spouse's doctor to see what the options are.

For men with PD, erectile dysfunction is common. Of course, erection problems are common in men anyway as they age, but men with PD can have even more trouble with this as the disease negatively impacts the central nervous system, circulation, and muscle function. Erectile dysfunction can affect self-esteem so it's important to be sensitive to that as well.

Women with PD may feel that their symptoms make them less attractive or desirable to their partner. Also, the hormone changes of menopause may contribute to some women having a decreased desire for sexual relationships.

Though it may seem less romantic, you might need to do a little planning before being physically intimate, or possibly consider different ways of doing so.

If your spouse has issues with erectile dysfunction, he may find certain medications helpful. Consult with the doctor to discuss possible drug treatments, as well as their potential side effects.

PART 7

Getting Help

40. Respite Care

"You need some alone time to recharge your batteries. Don't feel that you must carry this alone. Involve your family. Help each other. Being the caregiver is hard work. Don't be ashamed if you get tired. It is important that you talk to each other. Just because your mate has Parkinson's doesn't mean that they can't support you emotionally. It is the body that doesn't work, not the brain and heart!" —MELODY H., PARKINSON'S CAREGIVER

Respite is defined as "a short period of rest or relief from something difficult or unpleasant." If you plan on being a caregiver for any length of time, you will need this.

Respite care allows you to take a break from caregiving while someone else takes care of your loved one for a few hours, days, or weeks.

You may hear some people saying that you're "running away," but you're not. You're just stepping off the playing field for a little bit and giving yourself a break. This can also be a good break for your loved one with PD.

As the needs of the care receiver will vary, so will the amount of time off a caregiver will need. Depending on how much care your loved one needs daily, you may find that taking a few 15- to 20-minute breaks throughout the day is enough. Some caregivers need more than this, however, and choose to take one or multiple days off a week to avoid burnout.

Remember, as a caregiver it's essential that you not feel guilty about wanting to have time off and have a respite worker come in. It's not selfish for you to want this time off. Instead, it is absolutely necessary that you take it, for both your sake and the sake of the person for whom you are caring.

Help can come from many people, including friends, family, neighbors, or respite workers from local organizations. A respite worker is someone who comes into your home and helps a person with PD with activities of daily living, cooking, house cleaning, and so forth. When looking for formal respite care in your community, you should find several types available. These include companions, homemakers, home care aides, home health aides, adult day care, and overnight care for a few days or longer in a facility such as a nursing home.

Following are two types of formal respite care that have proven themselves valuable to caregivers.

Adult day care

Many people think that adult day care is just a nicer way of describing what is essentially a nursing home. This is not true. Adult day care programs work to help people keep their independence longer by offering activities and services geared toward their needs, knowledge, abilities, and level of participation.

Following are some of the activities offered at adult day care centers.

- Arts and crafts
- Exercise classes
- Musical entertainment and sing-alongs
- Mental stimulation games such as bingo and board games
- Discussion groups (books, films, current events)
- Holiday and birthday celebrations
- Local outings
- Occupational therapy
- Massage therapy

Adult day care programs are offered in a safe and secure environment, and most provide a light breakfast, lunch, and snacks. Some even have support and counseling services for caregivers and provide transportation to and from your home.

If your loved one needs extra care, supervision, or companionship during the day, or if you need respite during daytime hours, an adult day care center may be the solution for you.

The costs for these programs vary depending on where you live and what services they provide (e.g., meals, transportation, nursing supervision), but in the U.S. they average about $75 a day.[25]

Where there are professional health services, higher fees will apply. Some facilities offer their services on a sliding scale, meaning that what you pay is based on your income and ability to pay. Also, if your income is very low, Medicaid (U.S.) may pay for some or all of the costs.

You can find adult day care programs through your doctor or local aging society or by searching online for adult day care, aging services, or senior citizen's services.

Home care and home health care

Another popular formal respite choice is home care. You may have heard the terms "home care" and "home health care." The difference between the two is that home care involves care that is nonmedical and does not require a prescription, whereas home health care requires medical care and is prescribed by a doctor.

Both types of services are usually less expensive, more convenient, and just as effective as the care you would get in a skilled nursing facility.

There are many reasons you may want to use home care services as part of respite. One reason is for you to get relief from the more physically and emotionally draining caregiving tasks, such as bathing, toileting, and dressing. This will help prevent burnout. Another is having the convenience of being able to leave your home while the home care worker is there with your loved one, and having the choice to pay for only the hours or services you need (anywhere from a couple of hours to a whole day).

Your loved one may also appreciate home care if they have lost their ability to drive. A home care worker can provide transportation and accompany your loved to run errands or go to social events.

Finally, hiring a home care worker can give you peace of mind. Knowing that your loved one is getting the care they need when you're not there can really ease your worries. This type of care comes in handy if you live apart from your loved one and are caregiving from a distance.

Rates for home care vary depending on where you live and the amount of care you will need. You can find rates for the U.S. in chapter 8.

Following are some of the services provided by each type of home care.

Home care
- Personal care
- Dementia and Alzheimer's care
- Medication reminders
- Light housekeeping
- Meal preparation
- Transportation
- Grocery shopping
- Work in tandem with hospice and palliative care

Home health care
- Nursing
- Medication management
- Speech and language therapy
- Physical therapy
- Occupational therapy
- Wound care

If you live in the U.S. or Canada, an excellent online resource for finding home care is Senior Helpers. This organization has partnered with the Michael J. Fox Foundation to create home health care services specifically for people with Parkinson's. It also provides in-home services for those with Alzheimer's and dementia.

You can learn more about Senior Helpers by visiting https://www.seniorhelpers.com/ (U.S.) or http://www.seniorhelpers.ca/ (Canada). You can also find resources online by searching for home health care in your state or province.

If or when you decide to look for extra care inside your home there are several potential options, depending on how much care you want (visiting or live-in) and what kind of budget you have. Whatever type of caregiver you choose, you'll want to make sure you screen them by hiring a company to do a background check and to check their credentials.

One great feature of Senior Helpers is its Parkinson's Care Program. This specialized training program provides its caregivers with expert training and education necessary to create personalized care plans for individuals living with Parkinson's. You can learn more about it here: https://www.seniorhelpers.com/.

41. Housing Options

"My friend (with stage four PD) now goes to a day center twice a week where he has lunch and sometimes enjoys the mental exercise of an informal quiz afterward or recalling the words of an old song. He has home visits from the nurse on a regular basis, which is also helpful." —CHRISTINE, PARKINSON'S CAREGIVER

If you're new to the Parkinson's caregiving journey, where your loved one will live as their disease progresses may not be remotely on your mind. Or if you have thought about it there's been no question—they'll live with you at home!

Of course you may decide that your loved one will live with you for the duration of their disease, but for some who find the caregiving load in the later stages of Parkinson's to be too heavy, there are several alternatives to consider.

Before looking at the different types of senior housing available, it's a good idea to take stock of your loved one's care needs. Determining what daily activities they need help with will help you discern the type of housing that will best suit them.

There are two main categories of daily activities that aging adults (and, likewise, people with Parkinson's) typically need assistance with.

Instrumental activities of daily living (IADLs)

IADLs deal with the day-to-day maintenance of a person's environment.

- Cooking
- Doing laundry
- Housekeeping
- Driving
- Financial management

- Medication management
- Using the telephone

Basic activities of daily living (BADLs)

These activities involve attending to a person's hygiene, mobility, and bodily care needs.

- Bathing
- Dressing
- Toileting
- Eating
- Walking/getting up

Once you've discerned what activities your loved one needs help with, the next step is to learn about the various housing choices available. Many people get overwhelmed at this point, as there are many options. To make things easier, below I describe these choices and listed the pros and cons of each.

Living at home/aging in place

With living at home/aging in place, your loved one lives at home or with a close relative while their disease progresses. As mentioned in the previous chapter, adult day care centers can be a great option if your loved one is living at home, offering many activities for them while creating a caregiving break for you. Also, home care agencies can make things a lot more convenient for you by coming to your home and providing needed care for your loved one.

Pros
- Many aging adults feel best about living at home.
- Family members feel good about not putting their loved one in a nursing home.
- Care can be provided by either family members or home care professionals.

Cons

- Being the primary caregiver can be very emotionally, physically, and financially demanding.
- Caring for a loved one with Parkinson's can be a long journey, requiring you to give many years of your life.
- Relationships with your loved one may become strained.

If you're unsure about whether this type of care is for you and your loved one, asking yourself the following questions may help you decide.

1. Can your loved one's basic needs be met in the available space? The house may need to accommodate large assistive devices such as a lift chair, walker, wheelchair, bedside toilet, and so forth.
2. If you are the primary caregiver, do you work at home or need to be away from the home many hours during the day? If so, hiring outside help may be advisable. Someone must be available and willing to give medications at the scheduled times, prepare meals, assist with personal care, and provide transportation and companionship.
3. Do you have the physical and emotional strength to manage the care needs of your loved one yourself? If not, hiring outside help may be the best option for you.
4. Is the physical layout of the home user-friendly for your loved one? Doorway widths, stairs, and bathrooms are just three areas you will have to look at in your home to decide whether or not home care would be an option. There are modifications that should be made in advance to ensure the space is safe and comfortable (ramps at entryways, handrails, bathroom modifications, etc.).
5. Are there limitations such as young children in the home or lack of financial resources that need to be considered?

These could both contribute to a less-than-happy living environment.

6. Does your loved one want to live with family members, or would they prefer a formal care facility? Make sure you take into consideration your loved one's wishes.

Independent living/retirement community

Independent living communities offer various types of accommodations, from apartment-style living to freestanding homes.

Other names for independent living
- 55+ communities
- Active adult communities
- Adult lifestyle communities
- Life-lease communities
- Retirement homes
- Senior apartments
- Senior housing

Pro
- If your loved one is ready to move into a senior living community and is still able to care for themselves, an independent living community may provide the freedom and socialization they need.

Con
- Some communities provide assistance with certain BADLs (transportation, light housekeeping), but most aren't equipped to care for someone who needs extra help with bathing, dressing, and so forth.

Assisted living

Assisted living is good for those aging adults who want to keep their independence but who need help with some of their daily activities, such as meal preparation and/or bathing.

Assisted living accommodations include one-bedroom apartments, studios with or without kitchenettes, and single or shared rooms.

Other names for assisted living
- Congregate care
- Independent supportive living
- Retirement care
- Supportive housing

Pros
- If your loved one isn't safe living alone and needs only minimal assistance, assisted living may be a good option for them.
- Staff are available to help with IADLs, and medical professionals are there 24/7 in case your loved one's needs increase.

Cons
- As staff will be supervising your loved one when you're not there, the tradeoff is that your loved one will likely lose some of their overall sense of independence.
- The cost of assisted living does not normally include assistance with IADLs or BADLs. These services are available, but they will add to the price, so make sure you ask upfront what's included and what's not.

Skilled nursing facility (SNF)/nursing home

A skilled nursing facility/nursing home normally offers the highest level of care for aging adults outside of a hospital. They are designed for those who need around-the-clock, 24-hour care.

Pros
- SNFs/nursing homes have come a long way in recent years, and many are working hard to lose their negative image and to help elders live with dignity.
- The services of nurses, doctors, and physical, occupational, and speech therapists are all offered in SNFs/nursing homes.

Cons
- Your loved one may lose a lot of their freedom and independence.
- As a family member or caregiver, you may feel guilty for putting your loved one in a home.

Continuing care retirement community (CCRC)

The CCRC is a relatively new type of senior housing. It is designed to allow your loved one to remain within the same community but move into higher levels of care as their needs change.

Pros
- CCRCs may be a good option for your loved one if they want stability and security, as CCRCs take away a lot of the unknowns.
- Your loved one can more easily transition from one care level to the next without the stress or hassle of moving to an entirely new environment.
- There is a wide range of health care services provided, which may include nursing, doctor's care, social work, physical therapy, speech therapy, occupational therapy, a pharmacy, dietary assistance, and more.
- CCRCs offer many organized social and physical activities tailored to seniors' tastes. They are also most often situated in peaceful surroundings.

Cons

- CCRCs aren't cheap. Depending on where you live, this type of housing can be the most expensive long-term care option for your loved one. In most cases, residents are required to pay a large entrance fee, then a monthly fee after that. In some cases, residents buy the unit but still pay a monthly fee for services.
- It can be confusing to navigate the various types of complex contracts. It will be important to have an elder law attorney look over your contract to make sure you know what your loved one is signing up for.
- Administrators have the last word when it comes to when your loved one will move from one level of care to the next.

One question many of my readers ask regarding hiring in-home caregivers is whether they can help with giving medications. Home care workers can provide medication reminders and put the meds in your loved one's hands (provided that your loved one is aware they are taking meds). If your loved one can't put the meds in their mouth themselves, then the medication administration can be nurse-delegated to a qualified home health caregiver by a registered nurse (RN). If you are not sure what your loved one may need, check with their doctor.

42. When Is It Time to Apply for Disability?

"My advice would be just to take each day as it comes and enjoy the blessings around you. My husband continues to work and I believe that it is the best thing for him now. He is using his vast knowledge about his work and it continues to give him a sense of accomplishment. The people at his office are very supportive and caring." —JUDY, PARKINSON'S CAREGIVER

If your spouse or parent has Parkinson's and they are employed, how long they can work will most likely affect you as well. Because of this, the decision of whether or when to apply for disability is something you may want to discuss together so that you can be sure to make the right choice.

Because every case of Parkinson's is different, the decision won't be the same for everyone. If you live in the U.S., your loved one with PD will be eligible to file for disability benefits if they are unable to engage in substantial gainful activity (SGA) with earnings of $1,260 or more per month (the SGA level as of 2020).[26]

If you believe your loved one is disabled and unable to work and also believe that they may qualify for disability benefits, you should probably minimize the wait time by filing a Social Security disability insurance (SSDI) or Supplementary Security Income (SSI) application as soon as they are eligible. It is not uncommon for an application to take 6 to 8 months to complete despite the "estimated" 90 to 120 days that the Social Security Administration says it will take. (However, if your loved one's Parkinson's disability isn't obvious or doesn't show clear-cut long-term impairment, some disability attorneys suggest that they wait until they haven't worked for 6 months before they apply for benefits.) If your initial claim is denied, you will need to go through the appeal process, which adds even more time to the whole equation. Given these conditions, claimants for SSDI or SSI benefits often find themselves in great financial distress prior to a disability hearing.

The following links can give you more detailed information on applying for disability.

If you live in the U.S.: https://www.ssa.gov/disability/
If you live in Canada: https://www.canada.ca/en/services /benefits/disability.html
If you live in the U.K.: https://www.gov.uk /financial-help-disabled
If you live in Australia: https://www.australia.gov.au /information-and-services/benefits-and-payments /people-with-disability

43. How Can We Pay for Caregiving?

"Good luck to all who have this unfair card dealt their way in life. We have contacted a senior care advisor to get help with the finances and get the help we need to get him into a home. This has been our best call so far. They know all the hoops to jump through to get the most out of Medi-Cal and the VA. God be with all who have to deal with this."

—JACKIE W., PARKINSON'S CAREGIVER

We sold our family cottage on Canning Lake to pay for Mom's nursing home costs. My grandpa built the cottage, and all of us—Mom, her four kids, her grandkids, our cousins, even our second cousins—grew up having the most magical, never-ending summers there. It was such a special place. Our family had vowed to keep it in the family forever and never sell it . . . until we had to.

Losing the cottage was one of the biggest losses I've experienced in my life. First I was angry at Parkinson's for taking my mom from us, and then for taking our beloved cottage. Then I got angry at "the system" for requiring us to pay so much money for Mom to be taken care of.

If you've been on a Parkinson's journey with a loved one for any length of time, you may be able to relate to our story. At minimum you've probably had to look at your finances and financial future.

For the record, I want to say that although I was very sad about losing the cottage, in the end I was very thankful that we had an asset we could liquidate to pay for Mom's care. The money we made off the sale of that cottage was enough to cover about eight years of nursing home costs.

Another reason I'm thankful is that Mom lived in Canada, where nursing homes are considerably more affordable than they are in the

U.S. Wherever you live, it's a good idea to have a long-term plan to pay for care costs.

There are several avenues you can go down. To start, it is possible that your loved one will qualify for financial help from your government. It is very important that you investigate this to see if they qualify because there are many ways in which the government might be able to help you and your loved one. Depending on what country you live in, you may receive more or fewer benefits. Some governments provide help with buying things like wheelchair ramps or the funding for necessary home renovations to make things easier for people with disabilities. In most cases you would pay part of the cost and the government would pay the rest.

In addition, some governments (e.g., the U.S. federal government) have established or authorized some type of program to provide pharmaceutical (as in prescribed medication) coverage for low-income seniors or people with disabilities who do not qualify for Medicaid (U.S.) or its federal health benefits program.

Many governments will offer income tax relief to people with Parkinson's. You will need to fill out forms to apply for this, but it's worth checking into to see if your loved one qualifies for this. Sometimes, applying for benefits can be complicated, time-consuming, and frustrating. Two things you need to remember when going through this process are (1) do not throw away any potentially relevant paperwork you receive from an employer, an insurer, a government agency, or an advocate on your behalf and (2) keep copies of everything you submit.

Outside of government funding, there aren't a whole lot of organizations that provide straight cash. Well, not that I could find, anyway. (If you know of some, let me know!) One nongovernment organization I found that does help is the Melvin Weinstein Parkinson's Foundation. This a nonprofit organization dedicated to purchasing equipment and health supplies necessary to maintain a safe and healthy environment for Parkinson's patients. With the aid of support groups, the foundation locates Parkinson's patients who have financial and medical needs and finds a way to help them. To find out more, check out http://www.mwpf.org/.

Another possibility for financial assistance is through the World Parkinson's Program. This organization provides medications free of charge for people with Parkinson's who can't afford them. It also aims to provide assistive devices such as walkers, canes, and wheelchairs for free to those with PD who can't afford them. To find out more, check out https://www.pdprogram.org/.

The best way to receive monetary support is through either employment disability benefits or various federal health and/or disability support plans. If your loved one's income is low and they have few assets other than their home, they may be eligible for Medicaid (U.S.) health care coverage. This includes in-home care and personal care, such as help with bathing, dressing, cooking, cleaning, eating, moving around, and similar activities of daily living.

But before you do this, remember that there are planning options available to help you make the most of your assets. Consult an elder law attorney in your loved one's (U.S.) state. You can find one through the National Academy of Elder Law Attorneys. If possible, work with someone who is a certified elder law attorney (CELA). And remember that it's important to find an attorney you feel comfortable with.

Remember, you will need to do some research to find out whether your loved one qualifies for government assistance. You might start with your national Parkinson's foundation or society. You can find them online, and they can also direct you to your local chapter and they can tell you where you need to go.

Here are a few other online financial resources you may find helpful.

Paying for Senior Care (U.S.)
https://www.payingforseniorcare.com/

Medicaid (U.S.)
https://www.healthcare.gov/

https://www.healthcare.gov/medicaid-chip/getting
-medicaid-chip/

Benefits Checkup (U.S.)

https://www.benefitscheckup.org/. Benefits Checkup is the
nation's most comprehensive web-based service to screen
for benefits programs for seniors with limited income and
resources. It is provided by the National Council on Aging

Government benefits

In the U.S.: https://www.benefits.gov/. Benefits.gov is the offi-
cial benefits website of the U.S. government, with information on over 1,000 benefit and assistance programs

In Canada: https://www.canada.ca/en/services/benefits .html

In Australia: www.humanservices.gov.au/customer/subjects
/payments-older-australians

In the U.K.: https://www.careuk.com/care-homes
/choosing-funding-care/your-funding-options

National Academy of Elder Law Attorneys

https://www.naela.org/

44. How Do I Find Time for Me?

"Keep a strong body, mind, and soul. Make sure you take time out for yourself—maybe a trip to the gym or a good walk each day—at least 30 minutes. I do this very early in the morning before my husband is out of bed. We keep a positive approach to the situation, because there is always someone out there worse off than us. Make the most of the good days and the bad days won't seem quite so hard to take."

—HELEN G., PARKINSON'S CAREGIVER

Life as a caregiver can be so jam-packed, you may wonder how you could ever find extra time for yourself. This is especially true for those of you who are sandwich caregivers, juggling the care of your kids with the care of a parent with Parkinson's. Here's a ray of sunshine: caregivers who do find time for themselves end up with more energy and are better at stress management, enabling them to be better caregivers.

Most caregivers like the idea of "me time" but are convinced that they can't find it. You can! Believe it and bit by bit you will achieve it! Here are some strategies to help you find me time.

Schedule it

Many people use daily, weekly, and monthly planners and calendars to keep track of all their work and family tasks. Choose an organizational system that works best for you, then use it to schedule me time every day.

Even if it's only 15 minutes, include it in your daily to-do list and commit to making this time for yourself every day. You'll probably want to schedule this time early in the day so that other tasks don't bump it off the calendar.

If you are not used to making me time a priority, it may take you some time to get in the habit of doing so. That's why it's crucial that you schedule it and stick to it. Many professionals have said that it takes three weeks to build a new habit, so give yourself at least that amount of time to make this change.

Make sure you use your scheduled me time for something you enjoy, not for something like doing laundry or paying bills. Indulge in a nice cup of tea and a brand-new book. If you have a favorite art or craft (for me it's scrapbooking or oil painting), set up a craft table and have some fun!

In addition to your daily break, schedule a more substantial chunk of time once a week to do something for yourself away from home. This could include a spa day, shopping, or meeting up with friends for a movie.

Learn to say no

This is a tough one, I know. Though you may be able to say yes to most of your loved one's requests, there will be times when you need to say no, especially if they're asking you to take on a new task that would interfere with your own personal time (which is absolutely necessary for you to protect if you want to be an effective caregiver).

If you have a hard time saying no to your loved one's request, there are a couple strategies you can try. First, you can delay your answer. For example, you could say, "I'm not sure; let me get back to you." By answering this way, you give yourself time to think about whether the request is something you can or are willing to do. You will have to practice saying no and expressing regrets if you haven't done this much before. Don't worry. The more you do it, the easier it gets.

Another way to answer a request to which you want to say no, whether it be to your care receiver or anyone else, is by saying something like "I wish I could help but it will have to be another time," or "I'd love to help, but I just have too much going on right now."

Create a "me space"

Having a space in your home that is just for you can be a great way to get away while still being near your loved one if you need to be.

This personal retreat area can be something as simple as a comfy chair in a corner or a window nook. Or, if you have space, you can create a woman/man cave in a spare room or the garage.

Wherever you choose to create this personal space, make sure it's somewhere you can relax and be on your own (you may have to ask family members to respect your privacy when you're there). Decorate it with your favorite pictures and meaningful mementos, and stock it with anything you want to have nearby for your get-away (books, crafts, music, etc.).

Delegate or share tasks

To ensure you have the best chance of taking me time throughout your caregiving journey, minimize the time you spend on tasks that don't need your involvement. To do this, you will need to delegate or share responsibilities. For example, is there anyone in your household who could make dinner once a week? Could they do housecleaning or yard work? If you have kids, find things they may be able to help with. Consider making a chore schedule, with everyone in the household taking a shift.

As a caregiver, you may tend to help your loved one more than they need. Remember to let your loved one do the things they can still do for themselves. If they can still fold laundry or clean a sink (even if they don't perform the task as perfectly as you'd like), let them. This will help them feel useful and also free up your time.

Find shortcuts

One way to make time for yourself is to be more efficient. Spend a day analyzing how you do your routine tasks to see if you can save time. For example, schedule medical appointments first thing in the morning or right after lunch to avoid long waiting room times. Instead of going into your bank to pay bills, do your banking online. Run your errands when traffic is lightest and crowds are thinnest.

Another way to be more efficient is to multitask. For example, use Bluetooth in your car to make phone calls while driving to appointments or running errands. To catch up on your favorite prerecorded shows, watch them while you're getting your workout done on the treadmill.

If you can afford a laptop, iPad, or e-reader of some kind, these can be great investments for maximizing your time. You can use them while waiting for appointments, on the bus, or in between errands. These devices can be used to catch up on any work you have to do, or if you're in need of some me time, you can download your favorite books onto them instead of having to go to the library or bookstore.

Get unplugged

Here's a fairly easy way to make time for yourself: unplug for a bit. Almost all of us use electronic devices of some kind throughout the day, whether they are our phones, computers, or TVs. The question is, how much of that time is wisely spent? In other words, do you spend hours surfing the Internet aimlessly or reading and posting on Facebook, Twitter, or Instagram? Admittedly, it's nice to have electronics when you want to multitask (see above), but they can become dangerous time suckers if you aren't careful.

Start paying attention to how much time you spend plugged in every day. Consider taking a break from your devices, even if it's for only 20 minutes a day. See how it feels to be free of all electronics. You may find it easier to focus on your interactions with others and connect more deeply with them. You may also discover that you have a lot more free time for me time in a day than you initially thought.

Buy time

If you can afford to buy services to help make your life less burdened, busy, or chaotic, do it. This is one thing I've never heard someone say they regret. There are so many services available that can save you time and energy: housecleaning, grocery delivery, meal delivery, and yard work are just a few. And there are also the professional caregiving services, adult day care, and elder companion services discussed in chapter 40.

If you're not sure whether you want to spend the extra money on these kinds of services, consider how much of your valuable time will be saved by hiring someone to do these things.

To save money, consider paying a young relative or neighborhood kid to do yard work for you. You may be able to find help through local churches, Boy and Girl Scout troops, and schools as well.

If you have no extra money left at the end of each month, consider asking relatives who have offered help but who can't because they don't live nearby. Helping out financially could be an alternative way for them to reduce your caregiving load.

If and when you choose to buy yourself some time, do yourself a favor and spend that time on *you*. Though you may be tempted to run errands, aim to do something meaningful as well. Choose an activity that will nourish you so that you can come back to your caregiving tasks refreshed.

PART 8

Tough Caregiving Decisions and Issues

45. Decisions About Driving

"My aunt is 82 years old and lives next door to me. One of the most difficult parts of caring for my aunt has been . . . stopping her from driving. . . . In spite of all the reasons I gave her, she never quit arguing and begging until I told her, 'Continuing life without you would be unbearable for me. . . . I would not be able to forgive myself.' I explained that it wasn't because I thought she was incapable, but simply that her reflexes were delayed and would not allow her enough time to remove herself from danger. . . . Keeping her safe is my top priority."

—THERESA K., PARKINSON'S CAREGIVER

Many people think that once they have been diagnosed with Parkinson's they will have to give up driving. This isn't necessarily true. Each case of Parkinson's is unique, and the disease progresses at a different rate in each person. Although driving isn't safe in the advanced stages, people with milder symptoms who can control their motor movements can continue driving.

If you are the primary caregiver for someone with PD, it's important for you to know that there are several issues involved in deciding whether your loved one should be driving. Their physical ability, legal permission, safety, and the importance of keeping their independence are all factors.

Most likely, your loved one will be able to drive safely and legally for several years, depending on their age and general physical condition. However, PD and its medications eventually affect reaction time, ability to handle multiple tasks, vision, and judgment.

If you're thinking that driving may be a concern for your loved one, you'll want to ask yourself a few questions: Do they get lost frequently? Do other drivers honk at them? Do they have trouble staying in their own lane? If the answer to these is yes, it's time for them to give up their car keys.

If you do not feel that your loved one is safe, there are a few approaches you can take with them. First, you can take the direct approach: "Mom, do you think you should be driving anymore? It scares me to get in the car with you and I'm afraid you're going to hurt/kill someone." Another would be to call your local bureau of motor vehicles and express your concerns. They can have your loved one take a road test, which they will not be able to pass. Finally, you could ask their doctor to call and have their license revoked. In extreme circumstances, you may need to disconnect the vehicle battery and take away their keys.

My mom stopped driving about 15 years after her diagnosis because it caused her to tense up, and that caused her muscles to hurt. She also found her dyskinesia to be too much of an issue. She just felt safer having her husband drive.

46. How to Get Your Loved One to Consider Home Care

"Having different people come to the house, even for one to two hours, is incredibly helpful. The afflicted tend to become resentful of their caretakers, especially if they are family members. It is amazing how much more energy and motivation we see in my father when someone new shows up."

—KRISTEN K., PARKINSON'S CAREGIVER

If you've been caring for your loved one in your home for some time, or if your loved one lives alone but is no longer able to care for themselves adequately, you may have considered getting outside help.

Considering home care doesn't mean you don't want to be a caregiver anymore or that you don't love your spouse or family member; as the primary caregiver, it's your responsibility to keep your loved one safe, healthy, and properly cared for. Though your loved one may wish to live at home, they may not like the idea of having outside caregivers come into their house. You may need to help your loved one understand why they need help and why this option is best for you as well.

When you talk with your loved one about the possibility of choosing home care, make sure you listen to their thoughts and feelings. Put yourself in their shoes—it's not easy losing independence and freedom. Be sensitive and empathetic toward them. You might talk about burnout and how this will eventually happen to you if you don't get outside help. Let them know it will mean that you will no longer be able to care for them.

Next, explain why having some outside help could be a way to learn new things, as well as have some new company in the house for your loved one.

You might suggest a trial period so that both of you can see how and if this would be good for your situation. Remind your loved one that in the end, what helps you as the caregiver will also help them. Your loved one may need time to accept that they need help, so be patient and give them the time and space they need to come to terms with this.

If and when you decide to look for extra care inside your home, there are several potential options depending on how much care you want (visiting or live-in) and your budget. Make sure you do your homework first. You can hire help through a home health agency or hire a private caregiver directly, but know that there are potential disadvantages to the latter.

Following are some benefits of hiring a caregiver through an agency.

- The agency takes care of screening employees, doing background checks, and providing insurance, whereas private caregivers most likely won't have liability insurance or workers' compensation insurance, so you would be liable if an accident happened while they were working in your home. Also, if hiring a private caregiver, you would be responsible for filing tax forms and making sure they were eligible to legally work in the U.S. (or in the country in which you reside).
- The agency will send a backup caregiver if your regular caregiver is sick or on vacation.
- Agencies require a minimum amount of training (75 hours), whereas many private caregivers do not have formal training.

47. The Dreaded Nursing Home Decision

"To all caregivers of people with PD, please have patience. We do not want you to treat us like we're stupid. Don't treat us like we're kids. . . . We may be slower at doing things. I cannot write very well, I cannot write numbers, I cannot carry or pour. When we feed ourselves, don't laugh because we drop half our food down the front of ourselves, and please don't offer to buy us a bib! When you tell us something, don't get angry at us because we forgot what you said. HAVE PATIENCE AND UNDERSTANDING." —KATHLEEN, PWP

When Mom appointed me as power of attorney (POA) for her care, I was both honored and afraid. Honored that she felt she could entrust me to make sure she got the best possible quality of care and scared that it might be a tough thing to do. This appointment happened a few years before Mom developed dementia. Thankfully she had the forethought to do so, because it turns out that many care decisions need to be made when it comes to the later stages of Parkinson's disease.

When Mom gave me this mission, I told her I would do my utmost to make sure she would get the best quality of care and to live the best quality of life for as long as she possibly could. After all, Mom would have done nothing less for me.

When it came to the nursing home discussion, this is something Mom was able to have with her family before she developed dementia. Again, this was fortunate for us, as we could then feel less stress about making this hard decision.

We (Mom and her closest family members) made the decision together that she would try out a nursing home. Unfortunately, none of us was in the position to house Mom, let alone give her the around-the-clock care that she needed. Though it certainly wasn't an easy decision for any of us, over time we realized that a nursing home was the only choice we could have made for her.

Most people cringe at the thought of moving their loved one into a nursing home. This is understandable, given their not-so-wonderful reputation. However, there may come a point in your caregiving journey when your loved one's needs exceed the care you can give them and it becomes in their best interest to move them into a long-term care facility.

Of course every situation is different, so there's no definite answer as to when—or whether—you should move your loved one into a nursing home. If you're having a hard time with the nursing home decision, there are a few things you should remember. First, placing your loved one in a nursing home isn't mean or selfish. As I said above, it can be in the best interest of your loved one. Second, remember that it's the disease making it necessary for you to do this, *not* you failing at caregiving. Finally, know that you don't have to make this decision alone. Talking it over with your loved one's doctor, a minister, or a social worker can help you go through the decision-making process. This will take the burden off you and allow you to feel less alone in the process.

One of the positives that can come from placing your loved one in a nursing home is connection. Because you no longer have to take care of your loved one's physical needs, you can focus on loving them and connecting with them in more emotional ways.

Here's a little P.S. to this discussion. If you're not sure whether the timing is right or, if you want to delay placing your loved one in a nursing home, you may want to try adult day care. As discussed in chapter 40, adult day care can give you and your family respite during the day while allowing your loved one to have access to the services and care they need. This may be a great solution until your loved one's care needs increase.

48. Keeping Peace in the Family

"I found if my husband stays very active, he does better both physically and mentally. So I suggest not sitting around feeling sorry for oneself." —ANONYMOUS, PARKINSON'S CAREGIVER

Things can get a bit tricky with family as you get further down the road with Parkinson's. As with any chronic illness, when a loved one starts to show signs of needing more care, there are many issues for family members to discuss and numerous vital decisions that need to be made. Sometimes the severity of these decisions and their potential implications can cause very heated discussions within a family.

Depending on how big your family is, and how many people want to be involved in the caregiving process (even if it's not hands-on), having family meetings to discuss your loved one's care needs can be both practical and helpful.

Before you have these meetings, it's important to keep a few things in mind. First, know that it's not uncommon for family members to disagree over how a loved one should be cared for. Even the most harmonious siblings can become divided on various topics relating to their parents' care. The good news is that peace is possible throughout the process.

Try the following strategies to help keep the peace when discussing your loved one's care needs with family.

Plan ahead

Before you have your family meeting, you'll want to choose the right place for it. Whether it's physically in the same room or on a conference call using Skype or FaceTime, it's important that every member feels welcome and comfortable.

The next thing you'll want to do is have a few key points written down that you want to cover during the conversation. If applicable, bring an up-to-date medical report on your loved one, as well as a list of your loved one's wants and needs with regard to care and support from the family.

Some questions you may want to discuss are where your loved one will live (e.g., in their home, with another family member, in assisted living), how much their care will cost and how that cost will be covered, how much time each family member has to visit or care for your loved one, and what the primary caregiver needs in terms of assistance and support from the family.

Accept that not everyone may want to be involved

Understand that not everyone in your family may want to be involved in the planning of your loved one's care. Whatever their reasons for wanting to be excluded, it's essential to respect their decision. You don't have to agree with it, but it's helpful to try to be understanding. If you let resentment build up, it won't be good for anyone.

Consider outside help

Every family member should be allowed to express their thoughts and feelings without being criticized or interrupted. If you happen to be in one of those families that likes to talk over or yell and fight with each other, you may want to think about asking an objective third party to sit in on the meeting and help facilitate the conversation. A few people you could consider are a family friend, a social worker, or a pastor.

Identify caregiving roles and responsibilities

The roles and responsibilities of your family members will depend on their individual relationship with your loved one, how much time they have to give, and where they live.

For example, if your sister lives far away from your loved one, she won't be able to give hands-on care, but she may be able to take charge of setting up appointments or managing finances.

Don't worry if things don't go perfectly

Don't expect to solve every problem in one meeting. Some questions will inevitably go unanswered, and not all plans will work out the way you thought they would. If you can accept the fact that sometimes your family will disagree or fight, it will allow you to stay calm and steer the conversation back to the problem at hand if things get off track.

Get organized and keep others in the loop

When it comes to maintaining peace in a family, I've found that the best offense is defense. If you keep members informed and updated about your loved one's status and care, a lot of problems and confusion can be avoided. Come up with a strategy for keeping family members informed. If there are any unexpected changes or there's an emergency, consider setting up a phone tree to spread the word.

After you have a family meeting, consider writing down a summary of what you talked about, what decisions were made, and so forth and emailing it to all family members. Making a tentative schedule for your next family meeting to reevaluate your loved one's care is also a good idea as regular meetings can help prevent miscommunications.

49. Parkinson's and Dementia: Caregiving for a Double Diagnosis

"I purchased a baby video monitor to be used when my mother is napping. It is hard for her to talk loud enough to call for help. She also gets confused sometimes when she wakes so remembering to ring the bell we once had wasn't working. Now my dad can safely do other things in the kitchen and keep watch over her. He can even see when she opens her eyes and is ready for help sitting up. I bought the one that included two cameras and you can even hear and see in the dark. He appreciates this on those nights when he can't sleep and must get up and be in the other room." —LESLIE S., PARKINSON'S FAMILY MEMBER

It wasn't a huge surprise for my family to learn that after 22 years of living with Parkinson's, Mom started developing dementia as well. I had read the statistics in numerous places—it is estimated that anywhere from 50 to 80 percent of people with Parkinson's have Parkinson's disease dementia (PDD).[27] PDD is common in people with PD, though it's important to note that not everyone with PD will experience dementia. Generally, if a person with Parkinson's develops dementia, they do so after having lived with the disease for many years or even decades.

It's tough when a loved one is diagnosed with Parkinson's, and even more so when you get a double diagnosis of dementia. PDD is more difficult for caregivers than some of the other types of dementia like Alzheimer's because of the added impact of motor loss in Parkinson's. Though the disease is progressive it can last many years, so it is essential to educate yourself about the condition as well as the best ways to care for your loved one so that you can continue providing care for many years.

Who gets PDD?

Parkinson's patients who have hallucinations, mild cognitive impairment (MCI), excessive daytime sleepiness, and/or more severe motor control problems have the greatest risk of developing dementia.

Could my loved one's PDD be dementia with Lewy bodies instead?

There are two types of dementia associated with Parkinson's: PDD and dementia with Lewy bodies (DLB). These conditions are very similar in how they appear, both in person and when the affected brains are looked at under a microscope. The difference is in the timing.

PDD is diagnosed when a person with PD has had motor symptoms for a year or more before they develop dementia symptoms. DLB is diagnosed when a person develops dementia symptoms within a year or even before they develop motor symptoms of PD.

How is PDD diagnosed?

As with other types of dementia, there is no single test that tells us for sure that a person with Parkinson's has dementia. Doctors can, however, order an MRI or a CT scan of the brain to see whether some other structural changes or pathologies may be causing the symptoms. They will also look at a patient's medical history and results from a physical examination and memory tests to make their diagnosis.

How is PDD different from Alzheimer's?

There are some symptoms of Parkinson's dementia that may vary from those of Alzheimer's and other dementias. With PDD, people usually have major problems with attention, have a hard time making decisions, experience challenges with planning and reasoning, have slow thought processes, and encounter difficulties with memory retrieval.

In Alzheimer's disease, there is a great loss of memory and intellectual abilities. The memory problem is more often one of storing memories as opposed to retrieving them, as in PDD. People with PDD may also have more insight into the fact that they have a memory problem than do people with Alzheimer's disease.

What are the symptoms of Parkinson's dementia?

The following are the symptoms of Parkinson's dementia.

- Changes in memory, concentration, and judgment
- Trouble interpreting visual information
- Muffled speech
- Visual hallucinations
- Delusions, especially paranoid ideas
- Depression and lack of motivation
- Irritability/moodiness and anxiety
- Disorientation
- Sleep disturbances or excessive daytime fatigue

Tips for caring for someone with Parkinson's dementia

To help your loved one in the early stages of dementia, encourage them to do the following.

- Stay mentally active (e.g., card games, board games)
- Stay physically active (e.g., walking, stretching)
- Do things they enjoy (e.g., hobbies, shopping with you)
- Stay socially engaged
- Stay positive
- Get enough sleep
- Relax

Try these strategies to make caregiving tasks easier.

- Embrace their reality. It's okay to tell little fibs to your loved one (e.g., that their spouse is still alive, even if he or she isn't), as this will keep them happier.
- Stay on schedule to reduce confusion.

172

- Make sure all living areas are well lit to prevent falls.
- Remove anything (or anyone) that could overstimulate your loved one. We found that excessive noise agitated Mom, so we tried to keep her in quieter areas as much as possible.
- Make your loved one's living area wander-proof.
- If your loved one gets agitated, try to determine the source. Use distraction and redirection if you can't calm them down. When this happened with Mom, moving her to a different location often worked (e.g., moving her from her room to the living room). Treats can also be used as a distraction. In my mom's case, soft chocolate often worked.
- Keep lots of snacks handy as people with dementia often have a hard time explaining what they want.
- Play your loved one's favorite music whenever you can.
- Learn CPR and the Heimlich maneuver.
- Care for yourself by connecting with others and getting respite.

You may find attending a support group for Alzheimer's in addition to one for Parkinson's helpful. If getting out of the house is difficult, there are online communities and support groups (see the appendix for a list) that can help you cope with your daily challenges without having to leave your loved one's side.

Remember, the more help and support you can get, the longer you'll be able to care for your loved one and the better caregiver you'll be.

If you're concerned about placing your loved one in a long-term care facility, you may find it comforting to know that there are steps you can take to increase their quality of life while they're living in one, resulting in more peace of mind for you. You can find these in the resource section at AllAboutParkinsons.com.

50. Grieving While Your Loved One Is Still Alive

"Never underestimate how much of a difference you are making in your loved one's life. I cared for my mom with Parkinson's dementia for many years, and even in the late stages of her illness when she barely spoke, she would surprise me by saying 'I love you' out of the blue. Those three words meant the world to me." —ANONYMOUS, PARKINSON'S CAREGIVER

I don't talk a lot about Mom's last years of her life, mostly because I don't want to worry those who have loved ones with PD into thinking the one they care for will develop dementia as she did. As I mentioned in the previous chapter, not everyone with Parkinson's gets dementia. For those whose loved ones do experience dementia, however, I want to talk a bit about the grieving process that accompanies it.

For decades my mom and our family adjusted to the growing challenges of Parkinson's, and Mom did so like a champ. It wasn't easy by any means, but she kept on going, confronting each new battle head-on. When dementia started to creep in, however, it became quite tough for all of us to adjust to Mom's mind slowly dying.

I tried so hard not to say goodbye to her because I kept thinking, "She's still here! She's not gone yet!" For those who have never experienced dementia in their lives, it's tough to explain what it's like to lose someone who is still physically there. I have some very kind and well-wishing friends who would say that they were sorry about my mom having dementia but that I should be thankful she was still alive. I know they were right to some extent, but I wish they could have understood that though Mom was technically still living, she wasn't the same mom I used to know. She was a new mom that I had to get used to; my old mom was gone.

During my mom's dementia journey, I mourned many losses, and if your loved one has dementia, you will too. It's normal to experience a series of losses before the final goodbye and to grieve throughout the process.

You may find it weird talking about grieving when someone hasn't died yet, but psychologists say that grieving doesn't require a loss of life. They say that whether a person is still alive doesn't matter; the emotional process of grieving is the same.

If you're experiencing grief while caring for a loved one, the following are some ways to make life a bit easier.

- Be kind to yourself. Recognize that grieving can take a toll on your physical and emotional health. Allow yourself to take guilt-free breaks, be emotional when you need to be, and treat yourself to experiences that feed your mind and soul.
- Give yourself permission to live your life. This was a tough one for me, as I felt for a long time that my life needed to be on hold until my caregiving duties were done and Mom was gone. Over time I came to realize that Mom would want me to be happy and wouldn't want me to miss out on all that life has to offer.
- Slow down. Be present. Breathe. Caring for someone with dementia demands that you do these things.
- Reach out. Confide in other caregivers or support groups who know and understand what you're going through.
- Celebrate and cherish the memories you have with your loved one. Consider putting together an album (complete with photos and journal entries) commemorating their life story. If you have old family slides, you can have them transferred onto a DVD so that they can be enjoyed again.
- Get help from hospice care workers. They are trained to help those who have a life expectancy of less than 6 to 12 months and also work with families to help process grief.

If you have recently lost your loved one with Parkinson's, I'm deeply sorry for your loss. If you'd like to honor their memory, I invite you to have your loved one be a part of the Parkinson's Wall of Honor. For details, go to https://www.allaboutparkinsons.com/parkinsons -wall-of-honor/.

Acknowledgments

I want to express my sincerest gratitude to the Purdue University Press for helping me fine-tune this book so that it may help more Parkinson's caregivers. Thanks to their fantastic team, including Justin, Katherine, Kelley, and Bryan.

Thank you to my agent, Wendy Keller (Keller Media). Thanks for your patience in teaching me the ways of traditional publishing, and most importantly, for believing in me and my books.

Thank you to my editor and book coach, Kelsey Fritts. I'm so grateful for your insights and friendship.

A special thanks to Suzanne Newman (*Answers for Elders Radio*) for your friendship and support of this book. Thank you for your help in producing my Parkinson's podcasts and for having such a huge heart for our elders.

Thank you, Shawn D'Amelio, for introducing me to the world of home care and encouraging me to speak at conferences about caregiving for Parkinson's.

A big thank you to Mark Warenycia for all your work with AllAboutParkinsons.com and your continued support of all of its projects.

My deepest gratitude goes to all those who helped Mom live her best life with Parkinson's: To her sister Muriel, who cared tirelessly for her in her last two years of life and was there to hug her and hold her hand until the very end. To Mom's niece Shauna, for taking her on sunset walks and enjoying Cheezies talks with her. To the Lehto, Jouppi, Letourneau, Wagg, and Doherty families—I cannot thank you enough for the love you showed Mom throughout her illness. To Kate and Mignonette, thanks for all the care you gave Mom. Your extra special attention to her needs made a massive difference in her life. And finally, to Finlandia Nursing Home, for the exceptional care and respect you gave Mom in her last days. Thank you for allowing her to die with dignity.

An extra special merci beaucoup to my sister Tanya, whom I'll always call my twin because we're so close. Thanks for cheering me on and telling me I could do this author thing! Thanks to my sister Lara for being my inspiration every day and defying the odds of what can be done when one has advanced pancreatic cancer. To Brother T., aka my brother Tim, and sister-in-law Monica, thank you for your encouragement and prayers when I need them. To Maia and Ellie, thanks for being Gramma's little helpers.

My biggest thanks to my husband Nicholas. Everything I write comes from love, and your love keeps me going. Looking forward to many more books together!

My humble thanks to God, for blessing me over and over (and over) again. I am nothing without You.

Appendix

I'm very thankful that it didn't take long for my mom and stepdad to buy into the whole technology thing. Though there were learning curves, they found the benefits of having computers, cell phones, and other techie gadgets in their lives well worth it.

Following are my top recommendations for gadgets for people with Parkinson's and their caregivers.

Fall detectors

If your loved one has problems with balance or extra-fragile bones, having a fall detector is very important. Some medical alert systems also come with automatic fall detection, which senses when an elderly person has fallen down. Though these types of systems usually cost more, they can be worth it, especially in certain situations. If a person falls and is unresponsive, the medical alert system will notify the call center automatically. Also, the latest technology provides gyroscopes that can sense dramatic changes in position and alert backup, even if the person is not conscious.

One fall detector option (available in the U.S.), which includes GPS tracking, is the Home & Away Elite by Medical Care Alert. You can find out more about it by going to their website: https://www.medicalcarealert.com/All-In-One-GPS-Medical-Alert-with-Fall-Detection-s/1863.html.

Home phone systems

If you don't need or wish to pay a monthly fee for a fall detector like the Home & Away Elite, there are many options out there for systems that can alert someone if your loved one is having an emergency at home. One system that has received a lot of attention is the Vtech Amplified Big-Button Phone Series. It is an all-in-one communications center that includes a corded base and cordless handset with large-text display, large amber-backlit buttons, and audio boost.

Other features include the answering machine's ability to play back messages in slow mode to make them easier to understand as well as voice dialing, which allows you to call up to 50 numbers stored in the system.

The best feature is the wearable home SOS pendant. This pendant acts like a mini–cordless phone you can wear around your neck. It comes with two programmable buttons so you can program one to call a caregiver and the other to call 911. To learn more, go to https://www.vtechphones.com/products/careline-senior-phones.

Adaptive clothing

One of my favorite companies for adaptive clothing is MagnaReady. It was founded by a woman who was inspired to create clothing for her husband who has Parkinson's. Their clothing features magnetic fastenings, making dressing a lot easier (and less stressful!) for both men and women. You can find out more about them through their website: https://www.magnaready.com/.

Grabbers and reachers

Although these aren't very high tech, they can be handy for day-to-day living. Having one of these long tools to act as a secure hand to help pick up stuff off the ground can help people with Parkinson's keep their independence and also reduce the risk of falling.

Stabilizing utensils

Liftware Steady is a computerized, stabilizing handle with attachments, including a spoon and fork, which can help reduce mild to medium tremors enough to make it easier for people with Parkinson's to eat. To learn more, go to https://www.liftware.com/.

No-spill cup

If your loved one has tremor, pain, weakness, or other challenges that stop them from drinking easily, they may find the handSteady cup a great relief. This lightweight cup has a rotatable handle and hidden lid to help people drink with fewer spills and more control. To learn more, go to https://handsteady.com/.

Essential tremor glove

The Steadi-One glove was designed to reduce hand tremors in essential tremor and Parkinson's disease. The glove is lightweight and allows for a full range of motion while resisting multiple tremor directions that are common with ET and PD. To learn more, go to https://www.steadiwear.com/.

Weighted and vibrating pens

Thixotropic makes pens that are both large and weighted, making it easier to write with a tremor.

In 2015, students in the UK developed a vibrating pen to help combat micrographia, the small or cramped handwriting that many people with Parkinson's struggle with. Keep an eye out for these to hit stores in the near future.

Handheld massagers

Pain often accompanies Parkinson's disease, so it's important to learn ways to manage or relieve it. Whether it be in the neck, shoulder, or leg, massage can help. If your loved one finds going to a registered massage therapist to be too costly, handheld massagers are a great alternative. There are many different kinds, ranging in price from $10 to $200. Check your local drug or department store. You can also find many options online.

Simple cell phones

If your loved one is intimidated by smartphones, you don't have to worry. There are other phones, like those made by Jitterbug, that are easy to use and serve many purposes, including acting as a medical alert system. Some of the key features of Jitterbug phones are big buttons with large, legible numbers (to make dialing easy), a backlit keypad to assist visibility in low-light areas, and a powerful speaker so that conversations are loud and clear. To learn more, go to https://www.jitterbugdirect.com/.

Automatic pill reminders

If you know much about Parkinson's medications, you know how important it is that your loved one take them as prescribed. Being on time is especially important, and to help with this there are various options for pill reminders on the market.

One of the more basic types of pill reminders is a pillbox that allows you to organize medications by day of the week and time of day. They need to be filled accurately at the beginning of the week, but after that the pills are easy to find and take.

There are also pillboxes that come with an alarm (MedCenter makes a good one), or if your loved one prefers, you can buy a digital watch with multiple alarms to remind them throughout the day to take their meds. MedCenter has a five-alarm sport watch made specifically for this. Visit https://www.medcentersystems.com/ for more information.

Voice recognition software

If your loved one has challenges with typing on the computer, one solution is voice recognition software. One we like is called the Dragon Home. Dragon quickly transcribes words into text three times faster than typing with up to 99 percent recognition accuracy. With this software, your loved one can dictate and send emails, surf the web, and more, all by voice.

Visit https://www.nuance.com/dragon/dragon-for-pc/home -edition.html for more information.

Skype and FaceTime

Most of you have probably heard of Skype by now. It's an awesome free online service that can make such a difference in the lives of family and friends. With a simple download to your computer, iPad, tablet, or smartphone, this service allows you to see and talk to another person in real time. If you have an Apple product (iPad, iPhone, Mac computer), FaceTime is also a great way to see your loved ones.

I set up Skype for my mom on her tablet, and we used it until she passed. It was a real godsend during the times that we had to be apart.

HELPFUL RESOURCES FOR PARKINSON'S CAREGIVERS

Caregiver organizations

- Caregiver Action Network
  https://caregiveraction.org/
- Family Caregiver Alliance
  https://www.caregiver.org/
- The National Alliance for Caregiving
  https://www.caregiving.org/

Alzheimer's and dementia caregiving

- Alzheimer's Association
  https://www.alz.org/help-support/caregiving

Online communities, support groups, and resources

- All About Parkinson's Facebook page
  https://www.facebook.com/AllAboutParkinsons/
- Parkinson's UK Helpline forum
  https://forum.parkinsons.org.uk/c/living-with-parkinsons
    /carers-friends-and-family

- Parkinson's Foundation caregiver resources
  https://www.parkinson.org/Living-with-Parkinsons
      /For-Caregivers/Caregiver-Resources
- Caring.com caregiver support and resources
  https://www.caring.com/caregivers/caregiver-support/
- Today's Caregiver local resources
  https://resources.caregiver.com/
- AgingCare caregiver forum
  https://www.agingcare.com/Caregiver-Forum

Parkinson's foundations

Find information, clinical trials, and financial aid.
- Parkinson's Foundation
  https://www.parkinson.org/
- The Michael J. Fox Foundation for Parkinson's Research
  https://www.michaeljfox.org/
- The Davis Phinney Foundation
  https://www.davisphinneyfoundation.org/

Nutrition for Parkinson's

Learn about specialized nutrition for PWP.
- Education is Medicine
  https://educationismedicine.com/

Physiotherapy and online coaching for Parkinson's

- Invigorate Physical Therapy and Wellness
  https://www.invigoratept.com/

Housing help

Find homes that provide dementia care near you.

For housing help in the U.S. and Canada
https://www.alzheimers.net/find-dementia-care/

For housing help in the U.K.
https://www.carehome.co.uk/
http://www.housingcare.org/elderly-uk-nursing-homes.aspx
https://www.ageuk.org.uk/information-advice/care
    /housing-options/
http://www.housingcare.org/elderly-uk-assisted-living-extra
    -care-housing.aspx

For housing help in Australia
https://www.villages.com.au/aged-care

Legal assistance
- National Academy of Elder Law Attorneys
  https://www.naela.org/

Notes

1. AARP, *2015 Report: Caregiving in the U.S.*, June 2015, https:// www.caregiving.org/wp-content/uploads/2015/05/2015_Care givingintheUS_Final-Report-June-4_WEB.pdf; "Caregivers in Canada, 2018," January 8, 2020, https://www150.statcan.gc.ca/n1 /daily-quotidien/200108/dq200108a-eng.htm; Carers UK, "Facts About Carers," August 2019, https://www.carersuk.org/images/Facts _about_Carers_2019.pdf; Carers Australia, "Statistics," accessed February 5, 2020, https://www.carersaustralia.com.au/about-carers /statistics/.
2. AARP, *2015 Report: Caregiving in the U.S.*
3. Ibid.
4. Richard Schulz and Jill Eden (eds.), "Family Caregiving Roles and Impacts," in *Families Caring for an Aging America* (Washington, DC: National Academies Press), https://www.ncbi.nlm.nih.gov/books /NBK396398/.
5. AARP, *2015 Report: Caregiving in the U.S.*
6. "Caregiver Health," Family Caregiver Alliance National Center on Caregiving, https://www.caregiver.org/caregiver-health.
7. Laura Dixon, "Family Caregiving in 2017: A Full-Time Unpaid Job for Many," https://www.caring.com/research/caregiving-in-2017.
8. MetLife, *The MetLife Study of Caregiving Costs to Working Caregivers: Double Jeopardy for Baby Boomers Caring for Their Parents*, June 2011, https://www.caregiving.org/wp-content/uploads/2011/06 /mmi-caregiving-costs-working-caregivers.pdf.
9. "Caregiver Statistics: Health, Technology, and Caregiving Resources," Family Caregiver Alliance National Center on Caregiving, https:// www.caregiver.org/.caregiver-statistics-health-technology-and -caregiving-resources.
10. "Cost of Care Survey 2019," Genworth, https://www.genworth.com /aging-and-you/finances/cost-of-care.html.

11. Marlo Sollitto, "Family Caregivers Bear the Burden of High Elder Care Costs," updated June 17, 2019, https://www.agingcare.com /articles/cost-of-caring-for-elderly-parents-could-be-next-financial -crisis-133369.htm.

12. Elissa S. Espel et al., "Accelerated Telomere Shortening in Response to Life Stress," *Proceedings of the National Academy of Sciences of the United States of America* 101, no. 49 (2004): 17312–15, https://doi .org/10.1073/pnas.0407162101.

13. Marc A. Russo, Danielle M. Santarelli, and Dean O'Rourke, "The Physiological Effects of Slow Breathing in the Healthy Human," *Breathe* 13 (2017): 298–309, https://doi.org/10.1183/20734735.009817.

14. Jongeun Yim, "Therapeutic Benefits of Laughter in Mental Health: A Theoretical Review, *Tohoku Journal of Experimental Medicine* 239, no. 3 (July 2016): 243–49, https://doi.org/10.1620/tjem.239.243.

15. "Depression: Overview and Its Role in Parkinson's Disease," Diseases and Conditions, Cleveland Clinic, updated September 30, 2015, https://my.clevelandclinic.org/health/diseases/9379-depression -overview-and-its-role-in-parkinsons-disease.

16. Michelle Barnhart, Lisa Peñaloza, "Who Are You Calling Old? Negotiating Old Age Identity in the Elderly Consumption Ensemble," *Journal of Consumer Research* 39, no. 6 (April 1, 2013): 1133–53, https://doi.org/10.1086/668536.

17. "Caregiver Statistics: Demographics," Family Caregiver Alliance: National Center on Caregiving, https://www.caregiver.org/caregiver -statistics-demographics.

18. "Parkinson's Outcomes Project," Parkinson's Foundation, https://www .parkinson.org/research/Parkinsons-Outcomes-Project.

19. "Parkinson's Disease Dementia," Types of Dementia, Alzheimer's Association, https://www.alz.org/alzheimers-dementia/what-is -dementia/types-of-dementia/parkinson-s-disease-dementia.

20. Shannon Robalino et al., "Effectiveness of Interventions Aimed at Improving Physical and Psychological Outcomes of Fall-Related Injuries in People With Dementia: A Narrative Systematic Review," *Systematic Reviews* 7, no. 31 (2018), https://doi.org/10.1186/s13

643-018-0697-6; "Choosing Wisely: Physical Restraints," American Academy of Nursing (2015), Rev. 10/14, https://www.aannet.org/initiatives/choosing-wisely/physical-restraints.

21. Laurie K. Mischley, *Naturopathic Medicine in PD: Research Update*, June 19, 2018, https://www.youtube.com/watch?v=FHb2b-joVko&t=615s.

22. AARP, *2015 Report: Caregiving in the U.S.*

23. Richard Schulz and Jill Eden (eds.), "Family Caregiving Roles and Impacts."

24. "Sleep Disorders in Parkinson's Disease: Diagnosis and Management," *Annals of Indian Academy of Neurology* 14, supplement 1 (July 2011): S18–20, https://www.ncbi.nlm.nih.gov/pmc/articles/PMC3152169/.

25. "Cost of Care Survey 2019," Genworth.

26. "Substantial Gainful Activity," Social Security Administration, https://www.ssa.gov/OACT/COLA/sga.html.

27. "Parkinson's Disease Dementia."